DK The British Medical Association

FAMILY DOCTOR GUIDE *to*

CORONARY
HEART DISEASE

DK The British Medical Association

CORONARY HEART DISEASE

DR. CHRIS DAVIDSON

MEDICAL EDITOR
DR. TONY SMITH

DORLING KINDERSLEY
LONDON • NEW YORK • SYDNEY • MOSCOW
www.dk.com

IMPORTANT

This book is not designed as a substitute for personal medical advice but as a supplement to that advice for the patient who wishes to understand more about his/her condition.

Before taking any form of treatment **YOU SHOULD ALWAYS CONSULT YOUR MEDICAL PRACTITIONER.**

In particular (without limit) you should note that advances in medical science occur rapidly and some of the information contained in this book about drugs and treatment may very soon be out of date.

PLEASE NOTE

The author regrets that he cannot enter into any correspondence with readers.

A DORLING KINDERSLEY BOOK
www.dk.com

Senior Editor Mary Lindsay
Senior Designer Sarah Hall
Production Assistant Elizabeth Cherry

Managing Editor Stephanie Jackson
Managing Art Editor Nigel Duffield

Produced for Dorling Kindersley Limited by
Design Revolution, Queens Park Villa,
30 West Drive, Brighton, East Sussex BN2 2GE
Editorial Director Ian Whitelaw
Art Director Fiona Roberts
Editor Julie Whitaker
Designer Vanessa Good

Published in Great Britain in 1999 by
Dorling Kindersley Limited,
9 Henrietta Street, London WC2E 8PS

2 4 6 8 10 9 7 5 3 1

A CIP catalogue record for this book is available from the British Library

ISBN 07513 0678 9

Reproduced by Colourscan, Singapore
Printed in Hong Kong by Wing King Tong

Contents

Introduction

This book is about coronary heart disease, or CHD for short. The coronary arteries are the small blood vessels that keep the heart muscle supplied with the oxygen and nutrients that it needs to work properly and remain healthy.

Disease of in the coronary arteries builds up over many years and can lead to angina, heart attacks and sudden death. Coronary heart disease is the most common single cause of death in the UK. Most people will know someone who has had a heart attack, often without any warning, but this was not always the case. CHD has become much more common over the last 50 years, and we know some of the important factors responsible for the increase.

This book aims to tell you more about this condition, what to do if you have coronary heart disease and what you can do to prevent it.

There are several terms used to describe coronary disease and its effects on the heart. Coronary heart disease (CHD) is the term used throughout this book, but others that you may hear doctors use are shown in the box on the following page.

Coronary artery disease can cause a range of different problems, all resulting from insufficient oxygen reaching the heart muscle. The most common of these are:

A HEALTHY HEART
Lifestyle factors such as exercise have an important effect on the heart. Regular aerobic exercise will help to keep your heart healthy.

7

Terms that Describe Heart Disease

As you can see from the list below, doctors use a variety of terms to describe heart disease and its effects on the heart. The term coronary heart disease (CHD) covers all of these.

CORONARY ARTERY DISEASE (CAD)	Disease of the coronary arteries themselves.
ISCHAEMIC HEART DISEASE (IHD)	Narrowing of the blood vessels results in ischaemia – that is, lack of blood supply to the heart muscle.
MYOCARDIAL INFARCTION (MI), CORONARY, CORONARY THROMBOSIS, HEART ATTACK	Death of heart muscle as a result of a blockage in the blood supply.

● **Angina** Chest pain when exercising; this can include everyday physical effort, not just activities such as aerobics or jogging. The pain gets better when you rest.

● **Heart attack (MI)** Severe chest pain resulting from death of an area of heart muscle when the blood supply is cut off completely.

Other conditions that are often result from CHD:

● **Heart failure** Breathlessness and swollen ankles that results when the heart cannot pump well enough to keep up with the body's demands.

● **Irregularities of heart rhythm (arrhythmias)** Irregular heart beats that can cause palpitations and breathlessness.

CHD is not the only disease affecting the heart, but it is by far the most common in western countries. Other heart problems include:

- **Congenital heart disease** Abnormalities of the heart that are present at birth, such as hole in the heart.
- **Cardiomyopathies** Diseases that primarily affect the heart muscle rather than the arteries.
- **Valvular heart disease** Damage to, or abnormalities of, any of the four valves that control blood flow in the heart.

WHO GETS HEART DISEASE?

The number of people who get coronary heart disease varies enormously from one country to another. We are all used to the idea that certain diseases are commoner in some countries than others, yet we do not usually see our own country in the same way. But if we were looking down on the Earth from another planet we would be as struck by the very high rates of heart disease in the British Isles as we might be by malaria in the Tropics. Unfortunately, in some parts of the UK we head the world league table, which is something that, as a nation, we cannot ignore.

In general, CHD is a disease of affluence. It is rare in the Tropics and developing countries, and is most common in northern Europe, North America and Australasia. It does seem to be related to lifestyle, because when people move from the developing countries to a more affluent culture they get CHD much more often than they would have done at home. For example, immigrants from the Indian subcontinent who come to the UK are even more likely to develop CHD than people who were born here.

THE LIFESTYLE LINK
People living in developing countries generally have a lower incidence of heart disease, but their risk increases if they move to a more affluent country.

CHD Death Rate in the World

Coronary heart disease is generally higher in the more affluent countries than in the developing nations. The death rates from CHD are shown below for a selection of countries. The rates are particularly high in the old Eastern bloc nations.

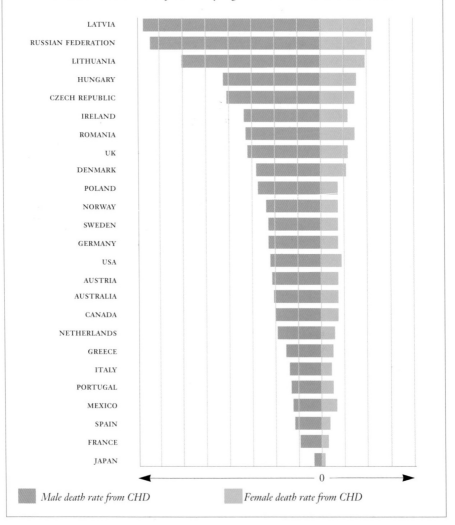

LATVIA
RUSSIAN FEDERATION
LITHUANIA
HUNGARY
CZECH REPUBLIC
IRELAND
ROMANIA
UK
DENMARK
POLAND
NORWAY
SWEDEN
GERMANY
USA
AUSTRIA
AUSTRALIA
CANADA
NETHERLANDS
GREECE
ITALY
PORTUGAL
MEXICO
SPAIN
FRANCE
JAPAN

0

Male death rate from CHD   *Female death rate from CHD*

Within Europe there are major differences between countries and even within one country. In southern Europe, CHD is generally much less common than in the UK and Scandinavia – one of the reasons for the popularity of the Mediterranean diet at present. Many people believe that this way of eating – with lots of fresh vegetables, salad, fruit, fish and relatively little red meat or dairy produce – can help protect against heart disease (see Diet, pp.84–86). In the UK itself there are also large variations between regions; the highest rates of CHD are in what were the old areas of industrialisation – northern England, Scotland, Wales and Northern Ireland.

Although descriptions of CHD date back to the classical world, it was not recognised to be a common disease until after World War II. Since then the rates, particularly among young men, have risen alarmingly. In the USA this rise peaked in 1970, and the rates have been falling steadily ever since.

The same fall has been seen in Australia and New Zealand, and now in the UK. Unfortunately, rates of CHD are actually rising rapidly at present in European countries from the old Eastern bloc, such as Russia and the Baltic states.

It is no exaggeration to say that most hospital beds in the UK are occupied by people whose illness is in some way related to hardening of the arteries, and the most common of these is CHD. Coronary heart disease is more common than all forms of cancer combined. It is

CHD AND DIET
A healthy diet that includes plenty of fresh vegetables and salad and is low in meat and dairy produce will help protect against heart disease.

11

more common in elderly people and four times more common in men than in women until old age. In young men it is the most common cause of death after accidents. Why is CHD so common in western countries? No one knows for sure, but diet, smoking, lack of exercise and social deprivation seem likely culprits. Of course these problems occur in other countries too, which is why there is so much focus on the British diet as the most likely cause. We shall be looking at these factors in more detail later.

NEW TREATMENTS

The last 10 years have seen enormous advances in the treatment of CHD. There are new drugs, such as the 'clot-busters' used after a heart attack, better drugs for angina and powerful cholesterol-lowering drugs, to name just a few. And we have come to understand the value of some of the older drugs, such as beta-blockers and aspirin. These can not only help in relieving symptoms such as pain; they can also slow down or even reverse some of the changes seen in the disease.

The biggest advances, however, have been in the use of surgery and angioplasty. Bypass surgery (CABG – often pronounced as 'cabbage' – which stands for coronary artery bypass graft) can transform the life of an angina sufferer and in some cases also reduces the risk of further heart attacks. Angioplasty – a technique in which tiny balloons are used to stretch narrowed or blocked arteries – can be very effective, especially now that fine wire stents (or internal supports) are used to keep the arteries open.

This is all good news for anyone who has heart trouble, but our priority should be to tackle the underlying reasons why CHD is so common and try to stop so many people getting it in the first place.

KEY POINTS

- CHD is one of the the most common causes of death in North America and western Europe.
- There has been an epidemic of CHD this century, which is now declining in North America and western Europe but is rising in countries in eastern Europe.
- New treatments, including bypass surgery, have helped considerably, but prevention remains better than cure.

What goes wrong?

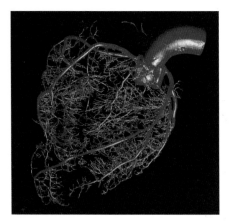

The heart is a muscular pump in the chest that is constantly working, pumping blood around your body, day and night, from the cradle to the grave. It contracts and relaxes 100,000 times a day, and all of this work needs a good blood supply of its own – which is provided by the coronary arteries.

CORONARY ARTERIES
This resin cast shows the system of arteries that brings blood to the heart. They supply the heart muscles with vital oxygenated blood.

HOW THE HEART WORKS

The basic function of the heart is to pump red blood, which is rich in oxygen and nutrients, though large arteries to the rest of the body. When the oxygen has been extracted by the tissues, veins carry the blood, which is now blue and low in oxygen back to the heart.

There are two sides to the heart, each of which acts as a separate pump. The two halves are sub-divided into two chambers, so there are four chambers in all. The upper ones, the atria, act as collecting reservoirs, and the lower ones, the ventricles, contract to pump the blood on. The right side of the heart receives blood through veins coming from all over the body and pumps it through the lungs so that it can pick up oxygen. The left side collects blood returning from the lungs and pumps it round the body to the tissues, which need oxygen.

The Internal Structure of the Heart

This diagram shows the two pairs of chambers – the left and right atrium and ventricle. Each pair acts as a separate pump. A valve at the exit of each chamber prevents blood from flowing back in the wrong direction.

Aortic arch

Pulmonary artery

Superior vena cava

Pulmonary valve

Left atrium

Right atrium

Mitral valve

Tricuspid valve

Aortic valve

Right ventricle

Left ventricle

Inferior vena cava

Descending aorta

In order to reach all the different organs and muscles, blood has to be pumped at high pressure, as you will certainly know if you have ever cut an artery – the blood spurts everywhere! To do this the heart is very strong and, unlike the muscles in our legs, for example, it doesn't become fatigued. The heart muscle does, therefore, require a very good blood supply, and this is provided by the coronary arteries and their branches.

How Blood Circulates Around the Body

Deoxygenated blood from the body organs and tissues enters the right hand side of the heart and is pumped to the lungs, where it takes up oxygen. Entering the left hand side of the heart, the oxygenated blood is then pumped to all parts of the body

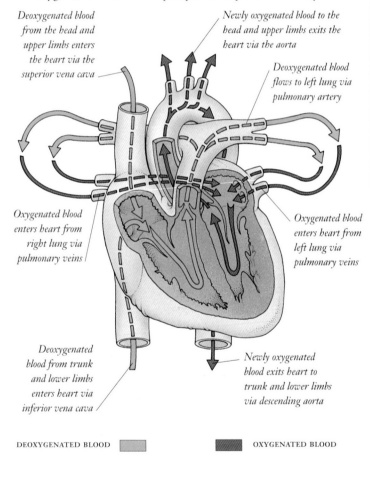

Deoxygenated blood from the head and upper limbs enters the heart via the superior vena cava

Newly oxygenated blood to the head and upper limbs exits the heart via the aorta

Deoxygenated blood flows to left lung via pulmonary artery

Oxygenated blood enters heart from right lung via pulmonary veins

Oxygenated blood enters heart from left lung via pulmonary veins

Deoxygenated blood from trunk and lower limbs enters heart via inferior vena cava

Newly oxygenated blood exits heart to trunk and lower limbs via descending aorta

DEOXYGENATED BLOOD   OXYGENATED BLOOD

THE CORONARY ARTERIES

The coronary arteries come off the aorta – the main blood vessel from the heart – just as it leaves the pumping chamber, the left ventricle, so they are the first arteries to receive blood high in oxygen. The two coronary arteries, the right and the left, are relatively small, each being just 3–4 millimetres in diameter.

They pass over the surface of the heart, meeting each other at the back and almost forming a circle. When this pattern of blood vessels was first seen by the ancients, they

The Blood Supply to the Heart

The right and left coronary arteries arise from the beginning of the aortic arch. These two arteries then branch into smaller vessels that supply oxygenated blood to the muscles of the heart.

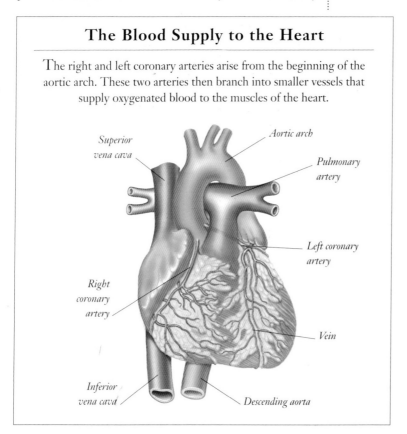

Superior vena cava

Aortic arch

Pulmonary artery

Left coronary artery

Right coronary artery

Vein

Inferior vena cava

Descending aorta

thought it looked like a crown and so they used the Latin name we have today, the coronary arteries.

As these arteries are so important, doctors are familiar with all their branches and the variations that can arise from one person to another. The left coronary artery has two main branches, called the anterior descending and the circumflex, which in turn have other branches of their own. It supplies most of the left ventricle, which is the more muscular of the two ventricles because it has to pump blood around the whole of the body. The right coronary artery is usually smaller and supplies the underside of the heart and the right ventricle, the chamber that pumps blood to the lungs.

The coronary arteries are similar in structure to all other arteries, but are different in one way – blood can only flow through these vessels into the heart muscle between beats, as it relaxes. While the heart muscle is contracting, the pressure is too great to allow any blood to pass through the heart muscle itself. This means that the heart requires a very efficient network of fine blood vessels within the heart muscle to get the blood where it is needed.

In CHD, the coronary arteries become narrowed (rather like a water pipe that becomes 'furred up'), and the heart muscle becomes starved of the blood and oxygen it needs. At rest this may not matter, but if your heart tries to work harder than normal – for example, if you walk up stairs – the coronary arteries may not be able to keep up with the demand for oxygen, and you get a pain in your chest (see p.39). If you rest for a while, the pain will usually go away. If a coronary artery becomes completely blocked by a blood clot, the area of the heart muscle that it serves will die (see pp.22–24).

ATHEROMA

Hardening of the arteries, atherosclerosis and atheroma are all the same thing. When you are born, your blood vessels are flexible and elastic and the blood can flow through them with ease. Early in adult life, however, fat deposits can start to form on the walls of the arteries. They gradually build up, forming lumps that protrude into the middle of the artery, and so reduce the blood flow.

The extent of these changes and the rate at which they occur are affected by the level of fats (technically called lipids) in the blood, especially one called low-density lipoprotein cholesterol, or LDL for short (see p.82). People who have high blood levels of LDL cholesterol are more likely to develop severe atheroma, but some changes may be present in all of us by the time we reach middle age.

As the patches of atheroma grow, they thicken and weaken the wall of the artery and progressively reduce the amount of blood that can flow through it. This process can affect any organ, so that atheroma of the arteries to the brain can lead to a stroke, to the limb, gangrene, and in the case of the heart, a heart attack.

The process of hardening of the arteries is curiously patchy throughout the body, and particularly so in the coronary arteries. The narrowing can just affect one coronary artery or part of one, or it can affect the artery throughout its length, and this may be important in deciding what treatment would suit you best.

In CHD, doctors often talk of one-, two- or three-vessel disease; this refers to whether the three main branches are affected, that is to say, the two main branches of the left coronary artery and the right coronary artery. In general, one- or two-vessel disease may be treated with medicines or angioplasty, whereas three-vessel disease, which affects all the major coronary arteries, usually requires bypass surgery.

THROMBOSIS

Thrombosis is the medical term for a clot, the natural process that comes into play to stop us bleeding when we injure ourselves. To stop the blood clotting at the wrong time, we also all have chemicals circulating in our blood that are natural anticoagulants or blood thinners. When a blood vessel is damaged, a whole series of chemicals is released close by, activating the blood and causing it to clot. In the case of coronary disease, a clot forms, not because of an outside injury, but as a result of damage to the lining of the artery caused by the fat that has built up in its wall.

Normally, the lining of our arteries is smooth and does not provide any focus on which a clot can form. When atheroma develops the lining is no longer smooth and, where there are breaks in the surface, small cells from the blood called platelets stick to these breaks and help to seal them. Providing the breaks are small, no harm results, but where the artery is critically narrowed even a small clot can have an important effect on blood flow. We now know that such a process is the cause of sudden deterioration in angina – so-called unstable angina (see p.40).

In a heart attack a rather different process is probably responsible. The fatty deposit in the artery does not just contain fat but is also surrounded by scar tissue caused by the cholesterol itself. This forms a fibrous cap over the top of the deposit that is much more rigid than the rest of

How Does Thrombosis Occur?

The process of thrombosis (blood clot formation) may be triggered by damage to the thickened lining of a blood vessel. The resulting clot may then obstruct the flow of blood through the vessel.

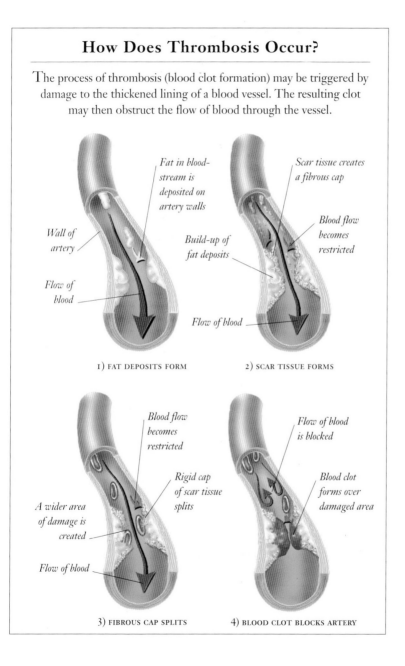

Fat in bloodstream is deposited on artery walls

Wall of artery

Flow of blood

Build-up of fat deposits

Flow of blood

1) FAT DEPOSITS FORM

Scar tissue creates a fibrous cap

Blood flow becomes restricted

Flow of blood

2) SCAR TISSUE FORMS

Blood flow becomes restricted

Rigid cap of scar tissue splits

A wider area of damage is created

Flow of blood

3) FIBROUS CAP SPLITS

Flow of blood is blocked

Blood clot forms over damaged area

4) BLOOD CLOT BLOCKS ARTERY

the artery. Any sudden stress can cause this cap to split, creating a wider area of damage to the wall of the artery. This results in a much larger clot forming, one that usually blocks the artery altogether. Blood cannot then reach the heart muscle beyond this clot and so that section of muscle dies.

Thrombosis, then, is one of the central problems in coronary heart disease. It is the cause of most cases of sudden deterioration in angina and of most heart attacks. As we shall see, the newer and highly effective treatments for coronary heart disease work by removing these clots and preventing their recurrence. We have complex and expensive drugs that can dissolve a clot in a heart attack, and simple, equally effective drugs such as aspirin that can prevent them forming in the first place.

We are trying to find out what factors make some people more likely to form blood clots than others. An increased tendency to clot may be one of the as yet undiscovered reasons why we in the UK are more susceptible to coronary heart disease.

HEART ATTACK

A heart attack is the final result when the diseased coronary artery becomes completely blocked by a clot, or thrombus. The heart muscle, or myocardium, beyond the clot is suddenly starved of blood and oxygen, and becomes painful, a pain that becomes more intense as the minutes pass. Unless the clot disperses by itself, which doesn't often happen, this area of heart muscle dies within 5–10 minutes, resulting in a fully blown heart attack, or myocardial infarction (MI) to give it its technical name.

The actual size of the heart attack and the amount of damaged muscle depends on a number of factors. The

What Happens in a Heart Attack

In a heart attack one of the coronary arteries suddenly becomes blocked by a blood clot, cutting off the vital blood supply to an area of the heart muscle.

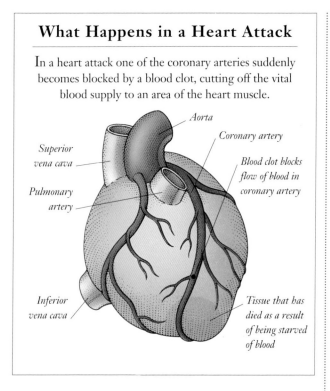

Aorta

Coronary artery

Superior vena cava

Blood clot blocks flow of blood in coronary artery

Pulmonary artery

Inferior vena cava

Tissue that has died as a result of being starved of blood

first is the size of the artery: the bigger the artery that is blocked the bigger the area of damage. The second is that the area of damage is generally greater when other coronary arteries are also diseased. Finally, the size of the heart attack depends on whether the area of muscle has developed any collateral blood supply (see p.25). If other collateral arteries have developed to supply the threatened area, the resultant damage is much less. Regular exercise is a good stimulus to the formation of collateral vessels, which is one reason why it forms such an important part of the treatment programmes of people with CHD.

The immediate effect of the damage to the muscle, apart from pain, is that the heart no longer pumps as effectively as before, and the blood pressure may fall, leading to faintness and sweating or nausea. The other major problem in the early stages is that the injury to the muscle causes irregularities of heart rhythm, or cardiac arrhythmias. These irregularities can be life-threatening and lead to a so-called cardiac arrest. As a result of the dangers of these arrhythmias, it is vital that the heart is monitored closely in the first 48 hours or so, and this is usually carried out in hospitals in cardiac care units (CCUs for short). Fortunately, such complications are rare after the first 2–3 days, and that is when most people can go to a general ward to recover before going home.

After a heart attack, the body begins to repair the damage straight away. Cells remove the dead or damaged muscle and fibrous or scar tissue is formed, a process that takes about 6–8 weeks. The scar itself is strong, but unfortunately the heart muscle that has been lost cannot be replaced and some weakening of the heart is an inevitable result. For most people with a small heart attack this makes very little difference to the overall performance of the heart as a pump. If a larger area of muscle is damaged, however, the heart becomes enlarged, and can no longer pump effectively, a condition we call heart failure.

THE END RESULT

Heart failure can be caused by many diseases affecting the heart, especially high blood pressure, but, in western countries, CHD is probably the most common cause. When the heart stops pumping properly, the lungs become congested with blood, leading to breathlessness. Congestion of the rest of the body also leads to fluid retention, which makes the ankles and legs swell. For many years the mainstay of treatment has been the drugs called diuretics or 'water tablets', which get rid of the excess fluid in the body and lungs. Now, however, we have a new class of drug called the ACE (angiotensin-converting enzyme) inhibitors that are even more effective, particularly in reducing the breathlessness.

The other result of the scarring of heart muscle is that it can interfere with the electrical processes responsible for maintaining the normal heart rhythm, and so lead to irregularities, or cardiac arrhythmias. The most common of these is called atrial fibrillation, which is usually treated with digoxin, an old drug derived from the foxglove. Other irregularities can be treated with drugs such as beta-blockers – one of the most useful drugs in CHD – and newer drugs are also now available.

COMMON FOXGLOVE
Digoxin, a well-established drug that is derived from the foxglove, is used to treat atrial fibrillation.

THE EFFECTS OF AGING

Coronary heart disease is a gradual and unpredictable condition. The fatty deposits in the arteries may build up very slowly over the course of 20–30 years. For most of this time there are no symptoms and angina only becomes a problem when one or more of the coronary arteries narrow by more than 70 per cent and blood flow to that part of the heart muscle becomes affected.

As the process is so slow the heart can find ways of overcoming the changes by developing new blood vessels called collaterals. The coronary arteries in effect form a network of blood vessels around the heart and, when one is narrowed, one of the other branches expands to help the area of heart muscle affected.

Although the build-up of coronary atheroma is slow, a clot can occur at any time. People who experience only occasional angina may get a sudden worsening of their condition – unstable angina – or develop a heart attack. Fortunately this doesn't happen very often; only about five per cent of people with angina per year experience such a deterioration.

What is much more worrying is the fact that a heart attack can occur 'out of the blue' in someone who has never been aware that he or she has a heart condition at all. This can happen because a relatively small fatty deposit, one that causes no real problem in terms of blood flow, can suddenly split and the clot that forms can block off the artery.

We are now beginning to understand this process rather better, and there are a number of drugs that seem able to stop it happening.

Case History 1: ANGINA

Three months ago, Arthur found he was getting a pain in his chest whenever he walked up stairs or when he walked up the hill to his home, especially on cold days. His GP told Arthur he had angina and started him on treatment with a regular anti-anginal medicine called atenolol. Arthur now feels well again and has no symptoms.

Case History 2: HEART ATTACK

John was a keen athlete and ran marathons. His father died of a heart attack (MI) when he was 64. John had been feeling quite well, but he collapsed with chest pain and died suddenly during a 10-mile run. A postmortem examination revealed that the cause of death was a heart attack.

KEY POINTS

- To function as a pump, the heart muscle is critically dependent on the coronary arteries for a good blood supply.
- In CHD, the coronary arteries become narrowed by fatty deposits or atheroma.
- Narrowing of the coronary arteries can starve the heart muscle of oxygen, and this results in the pain of angina.
- A heart attack results when a diseased coronary artery is blocked completely by a clot, and the heart muscle beyond can die.
- After a heart attack the damaged muscle heals by forming a scar; providing it is not too big, complete recovery can be expected.

Causes of CHD – why me?

There does not seem to be one single cause for coronary heart disease, or at least we have not yet found one. Medical research has, however, shown that a whole range of things can make you more likely to develop CHD, and these have been called risk factors.

CONSULTING YOUR GP
Regular check-ups are advisable if heart disease runs in your family, but there is much you can do to reduce the risk.

RISK FACTORS

Just as a tall person is more likely to hit his head on a door frame than a small one, so people with one or more risk factors are more likely to have a heart attack than those without any. However, not every tall person hits his head on a door and not every person with risk factors gets a heart attack, but the likelihood is greater.

The risk factors for heart disease are divided into those we can do something about – modifiable – and those we cannot – non-modifiable (see table on p.29). The risk of you or me developing CHD becomes greater the more risk factors we have, and these risks multiply together.

Not all risk factors are equal either. Some, such as smoking, can have a much greater effect on your chances of developing CHD. So, for example, a smoker with a high cholesterol level and high blood pressure has a much higher risk than if he or she had any of these factors by themselves.

However, a high cholesterol level by itself in someone who has no other risk factors means that the risk is increased to only slightly above average. This may well be nothing much to worry about; your doctor will be able to give you individual advice on this.

Factors that Contribute to the Risk of Developing CHD

MODIFIABLE	NON-MODIFIABLE
• Smoking	• Genetic factors, e.g., an inherited high cholesterol level
• Raised cholesterol	
• High blood pressure	• Gender – more men than women get CHD
• Diabetes	
• Obesity	• Age
• Stress	
• Lack of exercise	

Risk Factors that Affect CHD

Several factors have been found to influence an individual's risk of developing coronary heart disease. The greater the number of risk factors that apply to you, the greater your chance of developing CHD.

KEY:
HBP = HIGH BLOOD PRESSURE
RC = RAISED CHOLESTEROL

INCREASING RISK OF CHD →

						LACK OF EXERCISE
					STRESS	STRESS
				OBESITY	OBESITY	OBESITY
			DIABETES	DIABETES	DIABETES	DIABETES
		HBP	HBP	HBP	HBP	HBP
	RC	RC	RC	RC	RC	RC
SMOKING	SMOKING	SMOKING	SMOKING	SMOKING	SMOKING	SMOKING

RISK FACTORS →

AGE AND GENDER

Heart disease, like many other diseases, becomes more common the older we get. In the UK at present, half the heart attacks occur in people over the age of 65, and the numbers are rising as the average age of the population increases.

The striking thing about CHD is that, below the age of 55, it is a much more common disease among men than women. This is because, before the menopause (the change of life when women stop menstruating), women very rarely have heart attacks. After the menopause, CHD becomes more common so that the rate among women gradually catches up with men, and over the age of 75 the numbers are about equal.

The exact reason why women are protected from CHD before the menopause is not known for sure but it does seem likely that this is related to hormones that disappear once menstruation stops. Now that so many women are taking HRT (hormone replacement therapy) there is some evidence that this can protect against heart attacks and many doctors are recommending HRT for this reason (as well as, of course, for many others).

FAMILY HISTORY

Doctors talk about a positive family history when one or more close relatives (for example, parents, brothers, sisters or children) have had CHD. If your father suffered from a heart attack below the age of 60 or your mother below the age of 65, this increases your own risk of CHD. Of course, if your parents lived to an age when heart attacks become common, this is not so important.

WOMEN AND CHD
Post-menopausal women are just as likely as men to develop CHD. Before the menopause, hormones may offer women some form of protection, but the mechanism is not yet fully understood.

The same also applies to brothers and sisters, although, in very large families, the fact that one member may have a heart attack could be just the result of chance.

How is it that CHD runs in families? Part of the explanation lies in the genes that we inherit from our parents, which may make us more liable to have high cholesterol or develop high blood pressure or diabetes. Part of it is also the result of families living similar lifestyles – they all eat the same food and, if parents smoke, often their children do too.

If heart disease does appear to run in your family it is very useful to have check-ups from time to time with your doctor, to make sure that you have not developed high cholesterol, high blood pressure or any other problems that could be treated to reduce your risk.

RUNNING IN THE FAMILY
Heart disease may be common in a particular family because of genetic factors or because all its members share an unhealthy lifestyle.

DIET AND CHOLESTEROL

As we have already seen, atheroma is the major cause of coronary artery disease. Deposits of fat and, especially, of cholesterol, known as plaques, form in the walls of the arteries. This makes them narrower and so reduces blood flow. When the plaques split, a clot forms on the damaged area, stopping the blood reaching a part of the heart muscle. This is what happens in a heart attack. This whole process is more likely to happen (and to cause more damage if it does) in a person who has a high level of cholesterol in the blood.

Your genetic make-up is partly responsible for determining your cholesterol level. Some families carry genes for raised levels of various kinds of blood fats. This condition is called familial hyperlipidaemia or FH for short. However, diet also plays an important part in determining cholesterol levels. The more fats – particularly animal and dairy fat – you eat, the higher your cholesterol will be and the higher your risk of CHD (see diagram opposite). So it really is worth reducing the animal fat content in your diet (for more on this, see pp.84–86).

THE FRAMINGHAM STUDY

One of the first studies that linked high cholesterol with CHD was carried out after World War II in a small town near Boston, USA, called Framingham. All the residents were examined at yearly intervals to see whether or not they had developed CHD. A strong link with raised cholesterol was found early on – the higher the blood cholesterol, the higher the risk of developing a heart attack. The Framingham Study also showed the importance of the other risk factors such as smoking, high blood pressure and diabetes, and these various risk factors have been confirmed over a follow-up period of nearly 40 years since the study first started. The study is still continuing.

SMOKING

Cigarette smoking is strongly linked to the risk of CHD. Chemicals in cigarette smoke are absorbed into your bloodstream from the lungs and circulate around the body, affecting every cell. These chemicals make the blood vessels narrow temporarily. They also cause blood cells called platelets to become stickier, so increasing the chance of a clot forming.

Pipe and cigar smokers do not have the high risk of cigarette smokers but are still more likely to get CHD

SMOKING AND THE HEART
The more you smoke, the greater the risk of developing heart disease. However, it is never too late to stop smoking. Ex-smokers are less likely to suffer from heart disease than smokers.

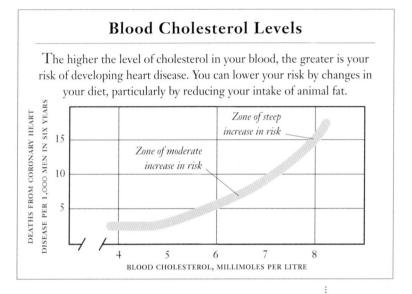

Blood Cholesterol Levels

The higher the level of cholesterol in your blood, the greater is your risk of developing heart disease. You can lower your risk by changes in your diet, particularly by reducing your intake of animal fat.

Zone of steep increase in risk

Zone of moderate increase in risk

DEATHS FROM CORONARY HEART DISEASE PER 1,000 MEN IN SIX YEARS

15

10

5

4   5   6   7   8

BLOOD CHOLESTEROL, MILLIMOLES PER LITRE

than non-smokers. The amount you smoke also matters; the risk rises stepwise between light (fewer than 10 cigarettes per day), moderate (10–20 cigarettes per day) and heavy smokers (more than 20 cigarettes per day).

The reason why doctors place such stress on stopping smoking is that it is the one risk factor that you can control yourself. What's more, you start to reap the benefit from the moment you stop. Although your risk of CHD may never be quite as low as that of a non-smoker, it certainly comes close to it a year or so after stopping.

STRESS

Many people who have had a heart attack point to some personal stress as a cause, but it has been surprisingly difficult to prove this link scientifically. There are well-recognised trigger factors, such as sudden unexpected exercise and extreme emotional experiences, which can bring on a heart attack, but this is a fairly rare occurrence. Indeed, at times of great civil and military stress, such as in World War II, the number of heart attacks in the civilian population actually fell.

We also often think of certain personality types as having a higher risk of heart disease than others. Modern technology has brought with it the ability to do things in an hour that even a generation ago might have taken days. The pressure to take on more than you can manage, to set unrealistic goals, has created the idea of the type A personality. This restless individual (usually male), who finds it difficult to relax, becomes increasingly tied up in work at the expense of personal relationships and is prone in the end to 'burn-out'; he is said to have double the risk of CHD compared with the 'laid-back' type B personality.

This theory linking CHD and the stressful personality was once very fashionable, and a lot of effort was devoted to trying to persuade people who had worked hard all their lives to relax. Modern research has failed to confirm these earlier findings and, although a major illness of any kind is a time to take stock of priorities in life, attempts to make major changes in behaviour are probably of little benefit.

— DISEASE LINKS TO CHD —

Two common and important diseases are associated with a higher than average risk of CHD: high blood pressure (BP) and diabetes.

- **High blood pressure** The term blood pressure actually means the pressure in the arteries taking blood from the heart to the rest of the body. High blood pressure causes

HIGH BLOOD PRESSURE
It is important to have your blood pressure checked regularly as high blood pressure can lead to damage in the arteries, increasing the risk of a heart attack.

The Sequence that Makes Up a Heartbeat

The heartbeat sequence has three phases – Diastole, atrial systole and ventricular systole. The timing of these phases must be accurately maintained, regardless of how slowly or rapidly the heart is beating.

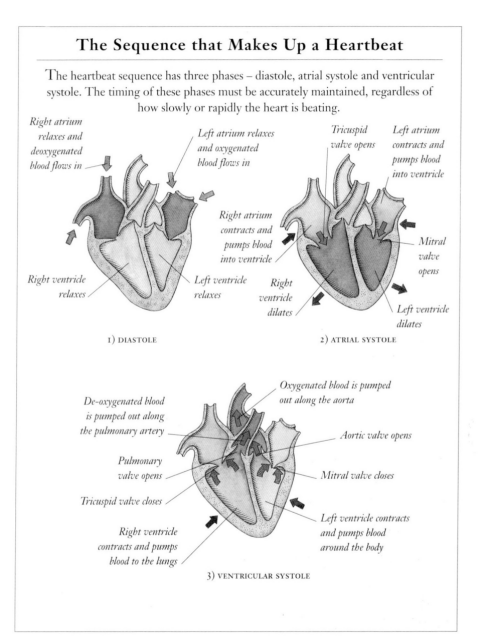

Right atrium relaxes and deoxygenated blood flows in

Left atrium relaxes and oxygenated blood flows in

Tricuspid valve opens

Left atrium contracts and pumps blood into ventricle

Right atrium contracts and pumps blood into ventricle

Mitral valve opens

Right ventricle relaxes

Left ventricle relaxes

Right ventricle dilates

Left ventricle dilates

1) DIASTOLE

2) ATRIAL SYSTOLE

De-oxygenated blood is pumped out along the pulmonary artery

Oxygenated blood is pumped out along the aorta

Aortic valve opens

Pulmonary valve opens

Mitral valve closes

Tricuspid valve closes

Right ventricle contracts and pumps blood to the lungs

Left ventricle contracts and pumps blood around the body

3) VENTRICULAR SYSTOLE

35

stresses on the heart and circulation and most people are aware that it causes strokes. However, in the UK high blood pressure is responsible for more heart attacks than strokes, probably because of the high cholesterol levels present in this country. Treatment of high blood pressure will reduce the risk of both heart attack and stroke.

Blood pressure is usually measured in the upper arm. With each beat of the heart, the blood pressure rises to a high point (systolic pressure) then falls to a low point between beats (diastolic pressure). This pressure is measured in millimetres of mercury (mmHg). An average healthy person's blood pressure at rest is around 120/70, said as 120 over 70. A resting pressure of 140/90 is borderline, whereas a resting pressure of 150/100 is definitely raised.

HYPERTENSION
High blood pressure is commonly found among Afro-Caribbean and black American people.

High blood pressure (or hypertension) is found right across the world and is particularly common in Afro-Caribbean countries and black Americans. It is also, however, very common in the UK, with perhaps 25 per cent of the population over the age of 50 having high blood pressure readings.

The cause of high blood pressure is not known in most people. It does run in families and is seen in people with kidney disease. Unfortunately, in most cases high blood pressure gives rise to no symptoms, and it is for this reason that it is sensible to have your blood pressure checked from time to time in case it is high and you don't know it.

The high pressure in the arteries damages the lining and accelerates the development of atheroma. The heart also has to work harder to pump blood under high pressure, but it must do so without an adequate supply of oxygen. This increases the person's chances of developing angina or having a heart attack. High blood pressure also increases the risk of a stroke because of the damage it causes to blood vessels in the brain.

- **Diabetes** This is a common condition that affects roughly three in 100 people in the UK. It is caused by a deficiency of, or a resistance to, the hormone insulin, which is essential to control the movement of glucose into cells around the body via the bloodstream.

Diabetes can affect people of any age, including children, and the younger you are, the more likely you are to need insulin injections to control it. Many people, however, get diabetes in middle or old age and, when this happens, there are few symptoms and the condition can be controlled by diet and tablets. The aim of treatment is to keep the level of glucose in the blood as close as possible to normal. Nevertheless, despite treatment, diabetes can increase the risk of many circulatory disorders including CHD. For women this is particularly important because it seems to counteract the protective effect of female hormones and almost as many women as men with diabetes develop CHD.

Good control of diabetes, with diet, tablets or insulin, makes heart and circulatory problems less common. Poor control can often result in very abnormal blood fat levels, including high cholesterol, and people with diabetes may need to take additional drugs to control this.

═ A WELL UNDERSTOOD DISEASE ═

But it is not all bad news. There are lifestyle factors that we can control that can reduce the risk of developing CHD and we will be looking at those on p.80.

People often feel guilty about having a heart disease, as if it is somehow their fault. That is not fair; the fact is simply that we know so much more about the factors that lead to CHD than we do about almost any other important disease.

KEY POINTS

- CHD is much more common in men than in women, and in the old than in the young.
- Important risk factors for CHD are smoking, raised blood cholesterol, high blood pressure and diabetes.
- Stopping smoking and reducing cholesterol and blood pressure levels cut the risk of CHD.

Recognising the symptoms

Although most people with CHD have the same underlying problem, namely narrowing of the coronary arteries, they don't all get the same symptoms. Some develop angina, others may have a heart attack. A smaller proportion of people may develop heart failure without having any previous warning symptoms. We don't know what determines these outcomes.

CHEST PAIN

Not all chest pain is caused by CHD. No one would think that they had heart disease after falling and bruising their ribs, for example, and most of us have had experience of painful indigestion, which can spread to the chest. You might think that it would be easy to distinguish chest pain caused by heart disease from any other kind of pain but in fact it can be difficult, even for the most experienced doctor.

● **Angina** *Angina pectoris* is simply the Latin for pain in the chest, and it is brought on by exercise, going away

A PAINFUL CHEST
Pain due to CHD is a dull, crushing feeling that usually starts in the centre of the chest and may spread to the neck and arms.

39

Exertion and Angina
Walking up a flight of stairs may be enough exercise to bring on the pain of angina.

when you rest. In CHD, the pain comes from the muscle fibres in the heart, which don't have enough oxygen for the work they are doing.

Angina usually lasts for about 2–3 minutes and no more than 10. It may only come on when you walk uphill, into a strong wind or when you're climbing stairs, but it can come on after quite mild exertion, such as getting dressed. It's usually worse in the cold weather and if you exercise after a meal – taking the dog for a walk after breakfast, for example.

● **Unstable angina** In general, angina is fairly predictable, but, if the coronary artery narrows still further or a clot forms on its surface, then the disease can enter a new phase – unstable angina. You may suddenly find that you can only walk a short distance before developing pain, or you may develop pain doing light work around the house or even going upstairs to bed. Sometimes you may be woken from sleep by an attack of angina. A change in the pattern of pain is an important development and should be reported to your doctor. Unstable angina can lead to a heart attack and it is important to take preventive steps.

● **Heart attack** The pain is the same as angina, but instead of easing off when you rest, it gets worse. People who've experienced it often say it's the worst pain they've ever felt in their lives. Someone who is having a heart attack may look grey and sweaty, and feel cold to the touch. They often feel sick and may vomit. Some people who have heart attacks have never had any symptoms of

How to Recognise Heart Pain

● A dull pain that does not feel worse when you breathe in.
● Usually in the middle of the chest but may spread into the left side, into both arms or up into the neck or jaw.
● Could be described as heavy, burning, vice-like or like a weight on the chest.

The Stages of Coronary Heart Disease

In a normal heart, the coronary arteries remain clear, providing the heart with adequate oxygen. A narrowed coronary artery will cause angina. When the coronary artery is blocked, a heart attack will result.

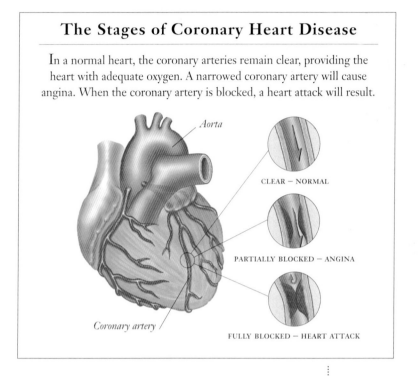

Aorta

CLEAR – NORMAL

PARTIALLY BLOCKED – ANGINA

Coronary artery

FULLY BLOCKED – HEART ATTACK

heart disease – it just comes out of the blue. However, most will have had some pain off and on for weeks or months before as the blood vessels gradually narrowed.

The difference between angina and a heart attack is that, whereas angina leaves the heart muscle short of oxygen but basically undamaged, in a heart attack a part of the heart muscle actually dies as a result of oxygen shortage.

In about 20 per cent of cases, the symptoms of a heart attack may be mild and are often mistaken for indigestion. This is particularly true of elderly people and those with diabetes, perhaps because the pain fibres to the heart are not as sensitive in these two groups of people.

OTHER CAUSES OF CHEST PAIN

We all experience various chest pains as we do in other parts of our body. Likely causes include the following:

INDIGESTION OR 'HEARTBURN'

The gullet (or oesophagus), which leads from the mouth to the stomach, lies just behind the heart and has the same nerve supply, so it is not surprising that pain from the gullet – heartburn – may feel much like pain from the heart. Heartburn can occur at any time but is usually related to food, starting half an hour or so after meals or when the stomach is empty. Heartburn can also occur at night when you lie flat because some of the acid from the stomach spills back into the gullet and irritates it. Eating more food or drinking milk or antacids eases heartburn, and hot fluids and alcohol make it worse.

Indigestion is not, however, brought on by exercise, and if you feel a pain in your chest when you walk – even if it makes you belch – it is much more likely to be from your heart than from your stomach. See your doctor.

PLEURISY

Chest infections such as pneumonia can give rise to quite bad chest pain called pleurisy. The pain is usually sharp, only on one side of the chest and is worse when you cough or take a deep breath. This is quite different from the dull constant pain from the heart, which spreads right across the chest.

MUSCLE PAIN

Along the back and between the ribs there are muscles that play an important part in breathing and, like all muscles, they can be subject to rheumatic pain. This pain

Other Types of Chest Pain

Chest pain can be alarming and often causes people to believe that they are having a heart attack. However, there are many other, less serious, causes of chest pain, including back injury and infection.

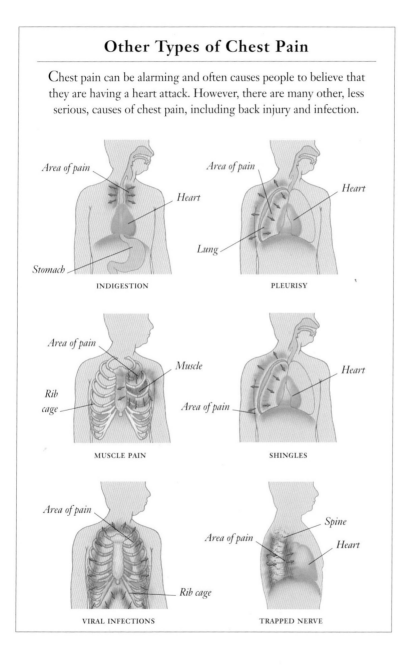

Area of pain / *Heart* / *Stomach*	*Area of pain* / *Heart* / *Lung*
INDIGESTION	**PLEURISY**
Area of pain / *Muscle* / *Rib cage*	*Heart* / *Area of pain*
MUSCLE PAIN	**SHINGLES**
Area of pain / *Rib cage*	*Spine* / *Heart* / *Area of pain*
VIRAL INFECTIONS	**TRAPPED NERVE**

is usually confined to a fairly small area of the chest, either at the front or at the back. It is worse when sitting or lying in certain positions or when you turn round. It can last from a few hours to a few days and then may disappear before returning again a few weeks later.

There are other possible causes of chest pain, although they are less common.

● **Shingles** This infection can cause severe pain around the chest for 2–3 days before the tell-tale blistering rash appears in the painful area.

● **Viral infections** Cold or flu-like viruses can affect the cartilage that attaches the ribs to the breastbone. When this happens, the chest will feel tender when you press it and the pain is quite different from heart pain.

● **Trapped nerve** Sometimes, pressure on a nerve in the back or neck can cause pain that spreads down the arm or around the chest. This can be caused by damage to a disc or by arthritis in the spine. Another relatively common cause, especially in women, is collapse of a bone in the spine. This is usually the result of osteoporosis, in which the bones become thin and fragile.

PALPITATIONS

Palpitations – when the heart beats irregularly or misses a beat – are very common in healthy people. They are usually brought on by stress, smoking or drinking too much coffee and tea. A few people may also have an electrical 'short circuit' in the heart that gives rise to a very rapid heart beat, but this is uncommon.

People with CHD can also develop problems with heart rhythm but this is most likely after a heart attack and your doctor will then give special drugs to try and control this. If your palpitations are associated with faintness, breathlessness or chest pain, you should tell your doctor as soon as possible.

BREATHLESSNESS

There are many possible reasons for breathlessness, of which the most common are probably chronic bronchitis, emphysema and asthma. Heart failure also causes breathlessness and can affect someone who has had a heart attack (see p.22). If the heart isn't pumping properly, fluid tends to build up in the tissues and lungs, and the result is breathlessness. You may then find it difficult to lie flat in bed or wake up in the night with problems getting your breath. You may also develop a cough with a little frothy or blood-stained sputum.

When fluid builds up elsewhere in the body, you may find your ankles swell or that you get pain in the stomach because your liver and gut are swollen. When you are known to have a heart condition, increasing breathlessness or a cough that won't go away may be important. There are now good drugs for treating heart failure and the sooner you seek help the better.

KEY POINTS

- When the heart muscle is short of oxygen, the result is chest pain – either angina or a heart attack.
- Severe chest pain is a heart attack until proved otherwise.
- Angina pain usually comes on when you exercise or are under stress.
- Indigestion is not usually brought on by exercise; if in doubt seek advice.

Tests for CHD

HAVING AN ECG
An electrocardiograph helps the doctor to investigate and diagnose a wide range of heart diseases. This simple test takes about 10 minutes.

There are many possible causes of chest pain, and the most important clue as to whether or not this pain is from the heart lies in what type of pain it is and when it comes on (see pp.39–44).

Doctors can usually distinguish between the different types of pain in the chest. It may become very clear, simply from what you are able to tell the doctor, that the pain is coming from your heart or that there is nothing to worry about.

The pain from a heart attack or from angina is often unmistakable. However, there are other times when the diagnosis is less clear-cut, and the doctor then has to make a decision based upon how likely it is that you might have CHD. In a young woman, chest pain is much more likely to be indigestion than angina, whereas in a middle-aged man who smokes and has high blood pressure it is more likely to be angina than indigestion.

Experience counts, but unfortunately no doctor is infallible, and many doctors have not even been able to diagnose their own heart attacks. But, because CHD is so common in the UK, most doctors will arrange further tests if there is any doubt about the diagnosis.

HEART TRACING

If heart disease is suspected, you will probably have a heart trace, known as an electrocardiogram. This test will record any abnormality in the electrical pathways of the heart.

RESTING ECG

The most common test for heart conditions is the electrocardiograph or ECG for short (in the US it is called the EKG). It is a simple, painless test that takes about 10 minutes and can be done by your doctor or practice nurse.

Every time the heart beats, it causes natural electrical changes that can be picked up by electrodes placed at various points around the body. These electrodes, covered in a sticky gel to ensure a good contact, are usually put on the ankles, wrists and across the chest.

The tracing records the heart rate and rhythm and whether the muscle is conducting electricity normally. Damaged muscle, or muscle that is short of oxygen, will result in a different appearance.

The resultant tracing gives the doctor a lot of information about the heart but, like most tests, the ECG is not infallible. Comparing the trace to normal ones or to one that you had taken previously will often show up a problem area.

If you have angina, your heart trace may still be normal if it is recorded at rest when free of pain. In this case, you may need an exercise ECG.

EXERCISE ECG

Any form of exercise can be used to provoke angina. In the UK, we generally use a treadmill test, but in Europe they often use a bicycle. ECG electrodes are attached just as for the resting ECG, but the wires are attached carefully to the chest so that they don't come loose while you are walking. The treadmill usually starts at a slow pace on the flat and then increases every 2–3 minutes to a faster speed on an increasing slope so that you are effectively walking uphill. The test is stopped if you develop pain, if there are major ECG changes or, of course, if you become tired or too breathless.

The useful thing about the exercise ECG is that it gives two pieces of information to the doctor. The first is that, if the test produces pain and ECG changes, it confirms the diagnosis of angina. The second is that, if you do well and manage to walk a fair distance before the pain comes on, it tells the doctor that the angina is mild and that further tests may not be necessary.

The test is usually done in a hospital and takes about 40 minutes.

EXERCISE ECG
Your doctor may perform this test to check the health of your heart. As you walk on a treadmill, your heart rate and the electrical activity of your heart are measured via electrodes.

RADIOACTIVE ISOTOPE TESTS

These tests make use of chemicals, or isotopes, that give out very small amounts of radioactivity that can be picked up by a special camera. Different tissues around the body take up different isotopes. For the heart various isotopes are used, the most common being thallium and technetium. Both these are taken up by heart muscle with a normal blood supply but would not be taken up by muscle that has a poor blood supply. So where there is a narrowing or blockage of a coronary artery, that area of heart muscle will not be seen as well as the rest of the heart.

Isotopes are, of course, radioactive, but the amount of radioactivity given in these tests is small and equivalent to most standard X-ray procedures. The isotope breaks down quickly in the body and some of it is passed in the urine, but it does not pose any danger to you or anybody else.

The isotope scan is carried out in two stages, once when the heart is stressed and once again when it is at rest, and the two images are compared. The stress pictures are usually taken after a treadmill test but, for those who can't exercise, the heart can be stimulated by drugs, the two most common being an injection of dipyridamole or dobutamine. At the end of the exercise test or after giving the drug, an injection of isotope is given and you then lie under the camera for 10–15 minutes while the pictures are taken.

ISOTOPE SCAN
In this coloured isotope scan of a normal human heart, the muscle around the left ventricle is seen as a blue/green arc. Areas of heart muscle with reduced blood supply can be detected by this method.

Sometimes, the isotope scan is better at picking up abnormalities than the exercise ECG, and it is useful after bypass surgery when the arterial supply to the heart can become quite complicated. It is also the only way to study the heart in people who can't manage the treadmill or bicycle, because of arthritis or bad lung disease, for example.

STRESS ECHOCARDIOGRAPHY

This is a new technique used in some centres that is similar in principle to the isotope test, except that radioactivity is not involved. Echocardiography is the name given to the scanner that uses sound beams to take pictures of the heart and is just the same as the ultrasound scanner used to see the baby in a mother's womb. With this type of scanner, it is possible to see the heart muscle contracting and to pick out any parts that are contracting poorly because the blood supply has been cut off. As in the isotope study, the heart can be stimulated either by exercise or by the injection of drugs and the heart is scanned before, during and after the stress. The pictures are then analysed in detail and can give good information as to which arteries may be blocked and how badly.

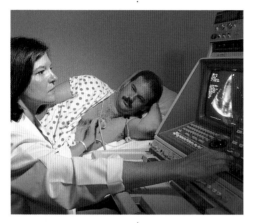

ECHOCARDIOGRAPHY
In this test, an instrument called a transducer, which produces a beam of sound waves, is held against the chest and directed towards the different parts of the heart.

CORONARY ANGIOGRAPHY

The most direct way of finding out what is wrong with the heart is to undertake special X-rays of the coronary arteries, called angiograms. These are X-rays in which dye that can be seen on an X-ray is injected directly into the coronary arteries. As the heart is moving all the time, the X-rays have to be taken on cine-film or video and it requires expensive equipment that at one time was only available in a few large teaching hospitals. With modern technology, these facilities are more widely available and most district hospitals can now undertake this test.

In order to take a picture of these small arteries, the dye needs to be injected directly into them. To do this, a fine tube called a catheter has to be passed to the heart, usually from an artery in the groin, but sometimes from an artery at the wrist or elbow. A little local anaesthetic is injected under the skin to numb it.

The catheter is then passed up through the artery towards the heart. You will not be aware of this happening, although when the tube reaches the heart you may have a few palpitations. This is quite normal.

Once the tube is in the coronary artery, dye is injected and pictures taken from various angles. While this is being done, you will be asked to hold your breath for perhaps 5–10 seconds. The dye itself may cause a little flushing that passes off quickly.

Coronary angiography is a safe and routine procedure. Serious complications are rare – less than one in 1,000. The most important risk, which fortunately is very rare, is that the investigation can provoke a heart attack. If this should happen, emergency surgery may be necessary. Less serious complications include an allergy to the dye or damage to the artery in the groin or at the wrist. Although coronary angiography is the best way of looking at the coronary arteries, it is not necessary for everyone with angina or CHD. Most doctors will use it only where they think there is a real possibility that you might benefit from heart surgery or angioplasty (see pp.58–63). Coronary angiography is often done as a day case procedure and takes about 40 minutes. You probably won't have to stay in hospital overnight but you will need to lie down for 3–4 hours afterwards to reduce the risk of any bleeding. The area used for the test will often be bruised and may be a little tender for a few days.

ANGIOGRAM OF THE HEART
This X-ray of the heart, taken after injecting the coronary arteries with a dye, gives a clear view of the arteries that supply the heart.

KEY POINTS

- The most common test for coronary heart disease is the ECG, but it is not infallible.
- If the resting ECG is normal, a treadmill exercise test is a good way to show angina and see how serious it is.
- For anyone who can't exercise, radioisotope testing or echocardiography may be used instead.
- Coronary angiography is the best way of identifying which arteries are affected, but is not needed by everyone with CHD.

Treating angina

Angina is pain in the chest caused by inadequate amounts of oxygen reaching the heart muscle. It usually comes on after exercise and disappears after you have rested for a few minutes. Unstable angina is when the condition gets rapidly worse so that eventually you are in pain even when resting. It may be a warning of an impending heart attack.

The doctor's aim when treating angina is to increase the amount you can do before pain starts and/or to relieve pain once it has started. Treatment may be with drugs, angioplasty or surgery.

TAKING ADVICE
It is important to follow any lifestyle changes that your doctor may suggest, including taking exercise or giving up smoking.

MEDICAL TREATMENTS

Usually drug treatment will be tried first. Drugs work by reducing the amount of oxygen needed by the heart muscle or increasing the blood flow to the heart, or both.

Whatever treatment your doctor starts you on, it is important that you work together as a partnership. You must take your medication as prescribed – in most cases, this is likely to be once or twice a day. You should also

COMMON SIDE-EFFECTS
One of the most common side-effects of taking glyceryl nitrate is a headache, which may occur as the pain from angina subsides.

Warning

IF THE CHEST PAIN IS STILL NO BETTER 10 MINUTES AFTER A SECOND DOSE OF GTN, YOU SHOULD SEEK IMMEDIATE MEDICAL HELP.

make any necessary adjustments to your lifestyle. This might mean giving up smoking, losing weight and taking more exercise. You will find more about this in the section beginning on p.80.

NITRATES

Nitrates in various forms have been used for angina for more than 100 years, and are the most common drugs used to relieve the pain of angina. Glyceryl trinitrate (or GTN for short) is absorbed very quickly through the lining of the mouth and is either taken as a small tablet under the tongue or as a spray. It opens up, or dilates, the coronary arteries and so improves the blood flow to the heart muscle in areas where the coronary arteries are narrowed.

Nitrates also dilate the arteries and veins throughout the body and this can lead to side-effects, particularly dizziness and headache. If you do feel dizzy after using GTN, sit or lie down for a few minutes and the effect will usually wear off. The headache that often occurs after using GTN is caused by the blood vessels to the brain dilating. It usually comes on within a minute or two of taking the nitrate and disappears quickly if you spit the tablet out.

People often find that the pain from angina starts to ease as the headache comes on. The effect of nitrates is so predictable in CHD that doctors often use this to tell whether your chest pain is really angina. This is fairly reliable, but pain from the gullet (oesophagus) can also sometimes be eased by GTN, which can be confusing.

Anyone who has angina should always keep their GTN tablets or spray with them wherever they are in case they get an unexpected attack of chest pain. However, if you have opened a bottle of tablets but not used any for a while, do keep an eye on the expiry date – GTN tablets will not work once the bottle has been open for more than six weeks. GTN works very quickly indeed, so if the pain has not settled within five minutes of taking the tablets, it may be developing into something more serious. Your doctor will probably advise you to wait for five minutes and if there is no improvement to take another dose.

Nitrates can be swallowed as a tablet but are not absorbed all that well from the stomach, which is why other, more effective ways of taking them have been developed. Some special formulations include a longer-acting tablet that can be left between the gums and the

The Effect of Nitrates on the Heart

In cases of angina, when the blood vessels supplying the heart are constricted, nitrates can be taken to dilate the blood vessels and increase the flow of blood to the heart. As more oxygen becomes available, the strain on the heart is reduced.

Coronary arteries are constricted

Nitrates dilate the coronary arteries

Heart muscle is starved of blood and oxygen

Normal blood supply returns to heart muscle

DURING AN ANGINA ATTACK

AFTER TAKING NITRATES

cheek for several hours (called buccal nitrate). There is even a skin patch containing GTN. This is a transparent plaster containing the drug that is absorbed slowly through the skin. It is left on for 18 hours and is usually removed at night. Your doctor may try several different nitrates to find out which suits you best.

BETA-BLOCKERS

Beta-blockers are a group of drugs that were discovered 30 years ago and were a major advance in the treatment of angina. They were called beta-blockers because they block the effects of adrenaline on so-called beta receptors in the heart, lungs and blood vessels. Their effect is to slow down the heart beat and reduce the blood pressure, particularly during exercise, so enabling the heart to undertake more work before angina comes on. People with angina usually find that they can walk further than they could before, and have to use their GTN less often. Sometimes, people find that their angina disappears altogether, though it would probably come on if they exercised hard enough.

Unfortunately, beta-blockers do not suit everybody. They cannot be given to people with bronchitis or asthma as they make breathing even more difficult. Other possible side-effects include cold hands and feet, aching in the leg muscles when walking, tiredness and, occasionally, impotence. There are, however, more than a dozen different beta-blockers available at present and often people find that one suits them better than another.

CALCIUM CHANNEL BLOCKERS

Calcium channel blockers slow down the rate at which calcium can enter body cells, particularly in the heart muscle and blood vessel walls. This group of drugs has been developed over the last 20 years; they act rather like nitrates by dilating the coronary arteries and improving the blood flow to the heart muscle. Like beta-blockers they increase the amount of exercise you can manage before getting angina though they do not slow the heart rate. As they act in a different way, they can be used with beta-blockers or nitrates as well as by themselves. The most common side-effects, as with nitrates, are headaches and dizziness. They can also cause swelling of the ankles and constipation.

ASPIRIN

Aspirin should be taken by everyone with angina, providing it does not upset them. It works by 'thinning' the blood so that it clots less easily. The danger for someone with angina is that a clot will form in any narrowed coronary artery and lead to a heart attack. By reducing the risk of clots forming, aspirin reduces the risk of a heart attack. The amount of aspirin needed to do this is only 75 milligrams a day – a quarter of an ordinary aspirin tablet or equivalent to the old Junior Aspirin. At this dose side-effects are rare but there are some people who are allergic to aspirin (often those with asthma) or who find it gives them indigestion and who therefore cannot take it. A new drug, clopidogrel, may provide an alternative.

OTHER DRUGS

Other drugs are being developed all the time for the treatment of angina and your doctor may wish to use one of these in your case, either because others have not worked or because they have had side-effects.

Nicorandil is one of these newer drugs and acts a bit like nitrates and calcium channel blockers to dilate the coronary arteries. It does so, however, by a different mechanism and may work when nitrates don't.

In some situations your doctor may also try warfarin, a drug that 'thins' the blood even more than aspirin. This can, like aspirin, reduce the risk of a heart attack and it may also help angina.

SURGICAL TREATMENTS

By no means everyone with angina will need an operation but, where the symptoms are becoming difficult to control with drugs, the results of surgery can be dramatic. An individual who has had angina for years, for example, can walk without difficulty again and some have even completed marathons! There are now many procedures that can be used to improve blood flow, either by bypassing arteries (coronary artery bypass surgery, or CABG) or by stretching them (coronary angioplasty, or PTCA).

Although both CABG and PTCA work well, they are not really a 'cure' in the sense that they do not get rid of the basic problem, which is the 'furring' up of the coronary arteries.

You still need to take all the steps necessary to prevent the arteries from deteriorating, either by changes in lifestyle such as stopping smoking, or with drugs such as those to lower cholesterol, and sometimes both (see pp.80–90).

ANGIOPLASTY

Angioplasty was first used about 20 years ago and involves stretching narrowed areas of blood vessels to improve blood flow. This is much quicker and easier than CABG but may be less reliable in the long term.

In principle, angioplasty is a technique whereby a long, thin balloon is passed across the narrowed region of a blood vessel, over a very fine guide wire. The balloon is then inflated at high pressure and stretches the artery, often splitting the fatty deposits in its wall. When the balloon is deflated and removed, the artery remains open.

The problem with coronary angioplasty is that, in about one in four people, the narrowing may come back within a few weeks or months – either the artery is not stretched far enough in the first place or inflammation sets in and the fat comes back. If this happens, a second angioplasty may well be successful. There has, however, been a big advance over the last few years with the use of coronary stents.

A stent is a fine wire mesh that is stretched over the balloon and, as the balloon is blown up, it stretches with the artery and remains there to hold it open once the balloon has been removed. This helps to reduce the risk of a recurrence.

Unfortunately, this exciting new technique is not suitable for everybody. It is best for people with one or two areas of narrowing in large arteries, and is really no good for those who have many small narrowing areas or narrowing in all three coronary arteries. In these cases bypass surgery is a better long-term solution.

HAVING AN ANGIOPLASTY

• The operation is usually done on an overnight basis – you go in in the morning and come home the next day. From your point of view, the procedure is exactly the same as having coronary angiography (see p.50).

• A deflated balloon is passed with a fine wire into narrowed areas of the blood vessels and then inflated.

How the Balloon Angioplasty Procedure Works

Angioplasty involves widening the affected artery by inserting a balloon along a guide wire and then inflating it at the site of the blockage. Sometimes a fine wire mesh stent is used to hold the artery open. This helps prevent any recurrence.

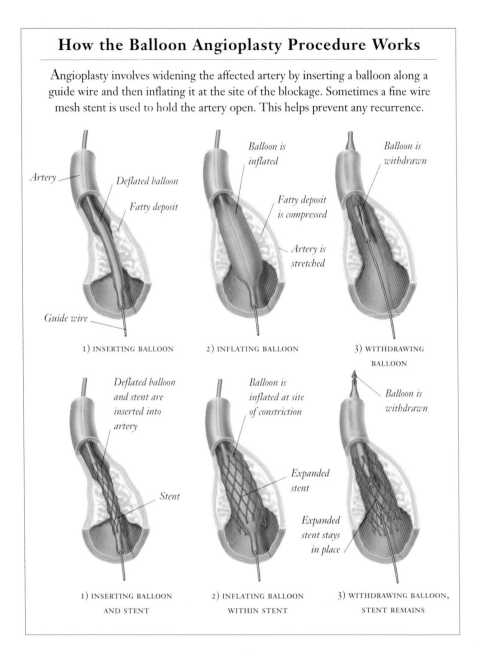

Artery

Deflated balloon

Fatty deposit

Guide wire

1) INSERTING BALLOON

Balloon is inflated

Fatty deposit is compressed

Artery is stretched

2) INFLATING BALLOON

Balloon is withdrawn

3) WITHDRAWING BALLOON

Deflated balloon and stent are inserted into artery

Stent

1) INSERTING BALLOON AND STENT

Balloon is inflated at site of constriction

Expanded stent

Expanded stent stays in place

2) INFLATING BALLOON WITHIN STENT

Balloon is withdrawn

3) WITHDRAWING BALLOON, STENT REMAINS

- It is then removed – and you won't have felt any of this happening. Sometimes you may experience some chest pain during the procedure and there is a 1–2 per cent chance that angioplasty may cause a sudden blockage, necessitating an emergency CABG. Usually, however, you'll be back to normal after a week.
- Angioplasty can be repeated later, more than once if necessary.

BYPASS SURGERY

Bypass surgery has been one of the major advances in the treatment of angina. The name derives from the effect of the operation, which is to bypass the blockages in the coronary arteries using replacement blood vessels taken from the chest wall or the legs. You may also hear the term 'bypass' used to mean the technique carried out by surgeons when they stop the heart and let the heart–lung machine take over the circulation during the operation.

When the operation was first performed surgeons used veins removed from the leg. These were cut into lengths of 4–5 inches (10–13 centimetres) and sewn between the blocked coronary arteries and the aorta (the main artery leading from the heart to the rest of the body).

In the last 10 years techniques have changed and, whenever possible, most surgeons now use small arteries rather than vein grafts. The long-term results of this technique appear to be better than with veins, which were never made to withstand the pressures normally present in the coronary arteries.

The two most commonly used arteries are the internal mammary arteries that run down behind the breast bone.

Coronary Artery Bypass

Narrow or blocked coronary arteries can be bypassed to restore blood flow to the heart muscle. The bypass may be an internal mammary artery or several vein grafts linking the aorta to the arteries beyond the blockages.

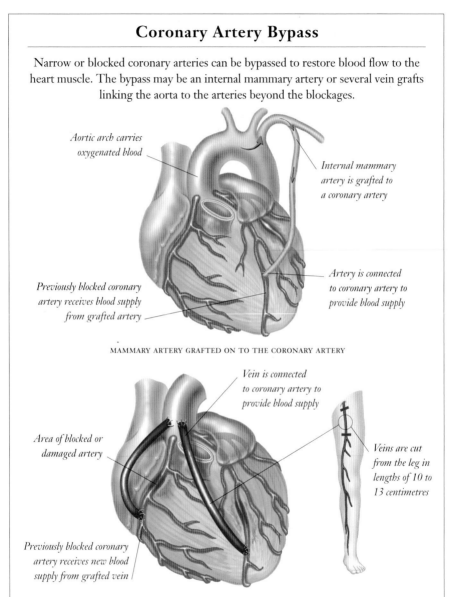

Aortic arch carries oxygenated blood

Internal mammary artery is grafted to a coronary artery

Previously blocked coronary artery receives blood supply from grafted artery

Artery is connected to coronary artery to provide blood supply

MAMMARY ARTERY GRAFTED ON TO THE CORONARY ARTERY

Vein is connected to coronary artery to provide blood supply

Area of blocked or damaged artery

Veins are cut from the leg in lengths of 10 to 13 centimetres

Previously blocked coronary artery receives new blood supply from grafted vein

VEINS ARE TAKEN FROM THE LEG AND GRAFTED ON TO THE CORONARY ARTERY

They can be attached to either the left or right coronary artery. More recently surgeons have even used arteries from the stomach or from the arm and both of these may last better than the vein grafts. Of course major heart surgery is not without risks and it would not be recommended for everyone with angina, particularly if the symptoms were mild. There are, however, some people with very few symptoms who may need bypass surgery because they have a high risk of a heart attack. This is usually because angiography has shown that all three coronary arteries are affected (see p.19).

A few people still have angina after CABG because it may not be possible to bypass all the blockages. Bypassing all the main arteries will reduce the risk of further heart attacks but some of the arteries may be too small to operate on, so mild angina may still occur, although it can often be controlled with drugs.

Unfortunately the new blood vessels may not last for ever and if they do narrow or block then a second operation may be needed. A second bypass can be more risky than the first, but using the new technique with mammary arteries, the long-term results can be just as good or even better.

HAVING A CABG

• Usually, you will be admitted to hospital for 1–2 days before your operation for final tests and assessment.

• On the day itself, you will go to sleep in the anaesthetic room and wake up in ITU (intensive care), probably still on a ventilator that is doing your breathing for you.

• You often have a lot of drips, drains and monitors for the first 24 hours or so, but after that most should be removed and you will go back to the ward.

• After 5–10 days, you'll be able to go home and, around 6–8 weeks later, you should be back to most of your normal activities. In other words, you can drive, go back to work (provided it doesn't involve heavy manual labour) and resume your sex life.

KEY POINTS

- Glyceryl trinitrate (GTN) taken as a tablet or spray under the tongue eases the pain of angina quickly, and should be carried at all times.
- Other drugs such as nitrates, beta-blockers and calcium channel blockers are very effective alone, and in combination, in controlling angina.
- Angioplasty (PTCA) is a technique where the narrowed artery is stretched by a high-pressure balloon, and is very effective in certain situations.
- Coronary bypass surgery (CABG) is very effective in relieving angina and is particularly suitable for advanced disease.

Treating a heart attack

If you have severe pain in the chest, feel cold, sweaty and nauseated, you are probably having a heart attack. This happens when a coronary artery becomes blocked, usually in an already narrowed artery.

The ambulance staff, paramedics, your doctor or a combination of all three may come to attend to you if you think you are having a heart attack, but their aims are the same – to stabilise your heart and reduce the amount of damage done to the muscle if it is at all possible.

When medical help arrives, you will be given oxygen via a face mask and have a plastic cannula (tube) inserted into a vein in your arm so that any drugs administered to you can go straight into your bloodstream. You will have ECG leads attached to your chest to monitor your heart rhythm, and you may be given morphine for the pain as well as something to stop the sickness.

EMERGENCY TREATMENT
A defibrillator is sometimes used to make the heart start beating normally. It works by administering an electrical shock to the heart via two metal plates that are placed on the patient's chest.

DISSOLVING THE CLOT

In the early stages after a heart attack, the most important early treatment is with drugs to dissolve the clot and, in some cases, this may be started before you reach hospital. Although it may sound strange, chewing on an aspirin tablet is a good way to start. It is absorbed through the lining of the mouth and starts to thin the blood immediately.

In addition to aspirin, we have many new drugs available. The last 10 years have seen a dramatic change in the way we treat heart attacks because we now have powerful drugs that dissolve the clot that is at the root of the problem. These drugs are called thrombolytics (though they are often referred to as 'clot-busters') and are administered by injection. The most common one used worldwide is streptokinase, but in some cases the more expensive tPa (tissue plasminogen activator) may be preferred.

The essential point about thrombolytics is that they work best if given within the first six hours after a heart attack. This is because, after this, the heart muscle may be too badly damaged even if the artery is unblocked again. Streptokinase is most effective if given in the first hour after a heart attack but it can still do some good up to 12 hours afterwards.

The use of these powerful drugs is not without some risk but large trials involving tens of thousands of patients with heart attacks have shown that the risks are greatly outweighed by the benefits. As thrombolytics dissolve

Treatment Priorities

The priorities of the medical care team in treating a heart attack patient are to:

- Relieve pain and other symptoms, such as nausea.
- Treat any serious cardiac irregularities promptly, with a defibrillator if necessary.
- Restore blood supply to the affected heart muscle by dissolving the clot in the coronary artery.
- Treat complications of the heart attack such as irregular heart beat or heart failure.

blood clots they do make people more liable to bleed. In some individuals, this may pose too great a risk – for instance, if someone has recently had a major operation, a stroke or a bleeding stomach ulcer – and in these situations other drugs may have to be given.

If you are given streptokinase, you will be given a card to show you have had it and when.

• This is because most people develop resistance to streptokinase after 5 days or so and this resistance lasts for a year or more.

• Therefore, if you need thrombolytic drugs within this period you will be given the alternative, tPa.

• It is very important that you carry this card with you at all times in case you are taken into hospital again.

REGULATING THE HEART BEAT

In the early stages, the damaged heart muscle can become very irritable and produce irregular heart rhythms, some of which can cause the heart to stop completely. Sadly, this is why some people die suddenly at home after developing chest pain before any help has arrived. These irregularities of heart rhythm – cardiac arrhythmias – can be treated very successfully by passing a brief electric shock through the heart using a gadget called a defibrillator – something you may well have seen on the TV or cinema screen. People who need this treatment have always lost consciousness, so an anaesthetic is not necessary. Unfortunately, the procedure only works if the shock can be given within a few minutes of the heart stopping, which is why the 999 ambulance and paramedic service are so vital. You may also be able to help if you know what to do (see p.91).

In hospital, people who have had a heart attack are usually treated in a special ward (the cardiac care unit) where the heart rhythms can be monitored closely for the first 24–48 hours – the danger period. If irregular rhythms start to develop they can usually be controlled with drug treatment and won't become severe enough to need a shock. After this the risk of rhythm problems becomes much less and drugs such as beta-blockers are used to prevent them happening again.

RECOVERING IN HOSPITAL

The worst period after a heart attack is the first day or two and, during this time, you will usually be monitored closely. After that most people have no more pain and are able to get up and about fairly quickly. After a straightforward heart attack, you may be able to go home after 5–7 days, but some people, particularly elderly people, may need to stay in hospital longer.

In the first week, although there is no more pain, you may feel tired and have a slight temperature, but this feeling usually settles as the healing process begins. The damaged area of heart muscle is repaired and a scar forms just like any other part of the body after an injury. This scarring is more or less complete 4–6 weeks after the heart attack.

If this is the first time you have been in hospital or had anything seriously wrong, it may take some time to come to terms with what has happened, especially if you have

STAYING IN HOSPITAL
Most people stay in hospital for about a week after a heart attack, although sometimes it may be necessary to stay longer.

financial and family commitments to worry about too. Nursing and medical staff are well aware of these worries and you should feel free to talk about them. It is time too to think about your lifestyle and what you can do to prevent another heart attack (see the section starting on p.80).

GOING HOME

After all the attention in hospital, it often feels strange to be going back home. You will naturally be worried about what you can and can't do, and your spouse or partner may be even more worried than you! In fact it is usually quite safe to do most things around the house, but any heavy physical activity should be avoided in the first few weeks. Remember that this includes some housework such as vacuum cleaning, which uses more energy than you might think.

It is very important in these early stages that your family and friends try not to be too overprotective towards you. For them and for you, every little twinge of pain may become larger than life, and most people after a heart attack become much more aware of aches and pains that they would previously have ignored. Indeed it has been reported that 90 per cent of people experience some form of non-cardiac pain in the first few weeks after a heart attack.

However, about one in three people get angina, which may feel similar to a heart attack. It will usually come on with effort, and ease when you rest. If so, you should take the GTN that you will have been given in hospital. If the

CAUSING CONCERN
The worry that friends and relatives will naturally feel must be kept in perspective. You need to take things easy without being over protected.

Drugs Your Doctor May Prescribe

After a heart attack your doctor will prescribe drugs to prevent a recurrence of the problem. This chart includes some of the more common drugs, but there are many other possibilities.

CLASS OF DRUG	GENERIC NAME*	ADMINISTRATION	PURPOSE	POSSIBLE SIDE-EFFECTS
Salicylates	Aspirin	Tablets	Thin blood	Gastric upset
Nitrates	Glyceryl trinitrate	Under the tongue, in the cheek, tablets, skin patches, ointment or spray	Relieve angina	Flushing, headache
	Isosorbide dinitrate	Tablets, capsules or under the tongue		
	Isosorbide mononitrate	Tablets or capsules		
	Pentaerythritol tetranitrate	Tablets		
Beta-blockers	Acebutolol	Tablets or capsules	Slow heart rate, protect against heart attack	Tiredness, lethargy, cold hands, nightmares
	Atenolol	Tablets or syrup		
	Bisoprolol	Tablets		
	Labetalol	Tablets		
	Metoprolol	Tablets		
	Nadolol	Tablets		
	Oxprenolol	Tablets		
	Pindolol	Tablets		
	Propranolol	Tablets or capsules		
	Timolol	Tablets		

Drugs Your Doctor May Prescribe (cont'd.)

CLASS OF DRUG	GENERIC NAME*	ADMINISTRATION	PURPOSE	POSSIBLE SIDE-EFFECTS
Calcium antagonists	Amlopidine	Tablets	Relieve angina	Flushing, headache, ankle swelling, constipation
	Diltiazem	Tablets or capsules		
	Felodipine	Tablets		
	Nicardipine	Capsules		
	Nifedipine	Tablets or capsules		
	Nisoldipine	Tablets		
	Verapamil	Tablets or capsules		
K+ channel activators	Nicorandil	Tablets	Relieve angina	Headache, dizziness, vomiting
ACE inhibitors	Captopril	Tablets	Protect against heart failure	Persistent dry cough, dizziness, occasional diarrhoea
	Cilazapril	Tablets		
	Enalapril	Tablets		
	Fosinopril	Tablets		
	Lisinopril	Tablets		
	Perindopril	Tablets		
	Ramipril	Capsules		
	Quinapril	Tablets		
	Trandolapril	Capsules		
Statins	Atorvastatin	Tablets	Reduce cholesterol	Headache, indigestion, occasionally muscle inflammation
	Cerivastatin sodium	Tablets		
	Fluvastatin	Capsules		
	Prevastatin	Tablets		
	Simvastatin	Tablets		

* *Pharmaceutical companies all give their products 'proprietary/trade' names as well as their actual 'generic/scientific' name. Only the generic names are listed here; you will be able to find this on the package of your medication.*

pain persists after using GTN, take another, and *if it lasts more than 20 minutes you should get immediate medical advice*. There may be a Helpline to the cardiac unit in your area and it is worth asking about this before you leave hospital.

TAKING MEDICINES AT HOME

During the first week in hospital you will be given a number of different drugs, some to treat complications and others to reduce the risk of further problems over the next weeks and months.

There is now a wide variety of drugs that may be given to people who have had a heart attack, and your doctor will decide which will do you the most good. Don't be surprised if you know someone who has been given different treatment as drugs must be tailored to suit the needs of each individual.

• **Aspirin** This is the most commonly prescribed drug, but some people can't take it, usually because they have stomach problems. Its main purpose is to reduce the stickiness of platelets – the cells in the blood that are involved in clotting.

• **Beta-blockers** These are drugs that block the effect of adrenaline on receptors in the heart and blood vessels, thus reducing the risk of another heart attack and cutting the death rate. Many physicians prescribe them routinely after a heart attack but some people can't take them, for example, if they have asthma, bronchitis or heart failure.

• **ACE inhibitors** These have been a major advance in the treatment of heart problems. ACE – angiotensin-converting enzyme – increases the amount of angiotensin in the circulation. Angiotensin makes the blood vessels constrict and causes the body to retain more salt and water than normal. ACE inhibitors, by reducing the angiotensin levels, have cut the number of people developing heart attacks and heart failure.

• **Statins** These are potent new drugs that lower cholesterol. They act by reducing the amount of cholesterol that is made in the body, particularly in the liver and help to prevent arteries furring up any further (see p.83).

• **GTN** This is one of the most important drugs you will be taking home, either as a spray or in tablet form. This is to use if you get any further pain in the chest after you leave hospital.

You should make sure you know how and when you should take GTN before you leave the hospital, and perhaps even try it so that you know what to expect. The doctors, nurses or pharmacist will answer your questions.

KEY POINTS

- Prompt treatment is vital. Call 999 rather than your GP.
- Close monitoring is required in the first few days, usually in a cardiac care unit (CCU).
- Most people can expect to recover fully from a heart attack in 6–8 weeks.
- Drugs are important to prevent a recurrence.

Getting over a heart attack

At one time doctors would have insisted that you stay in bed for around 6–8 weeks after a heart attack in the mistaken belief that this would allow the heart to heal better. It was not surprising, therefore, that after such a long period in bed that people felt worse than they did before they had the attack.

REHABILITATION

Rehabilitation after a heart attack is very different now from previously. Once the pain and general weakness have gone – usually a matter of a few days – the emphasis is on returning to normal over the next 6–8 weeks.

Most hospitals now have a cardiac rehabilitation service – 'rehab' for short. The aims of cardiac rehabilitation are:

- **Education** Understanding the cause of the problem and how you are going to get better.
- **Exercise** A graded exercise programme so that you can return to your normal activities.
- **Prevention** The steps you can take to avoid having a further heart attack.

EXERCISE AND THE HEART
A regular exercise programme is extremely important to maintain a healthy heart.

The rehab programme usually begins in hospital when a nurse will visit you and try to answer some of the questions that must be troubling you and your family. You should be given some guidance about what sort of things you can and can't do when you leave hospital.

The exercise programme usually starts 2–4 weeks later and is supervised by a physiotherapist in the hospital gym. There will probably be a group of 10–15 other people going through the programme and it is a good time to talk together and share experiences. It is often very reassuring to see someone exercising quite energetically as they come to the end of the programme when you are just starting and worried about doing any exercise at all.

For many middle-aged people, this may be the first regular exercise they have done for years and so it will seem strange at first. However, most people find the exercise becomes easier and easier as the weeks go by and are likely to feel fitter at the end of the programme than they have done for years.

Rehabilitation sessions usually last 1–2 hours and take place about twice a week for 6–8 weeks. As well as the exercise itself there is usually time to have some discussion about the cause of heart attacks and what can be done to prevent them. There may also be visits from a pharmacist, a dietician and a cardiologist to answer any questions you or your partner may have about your condition.

RETURNING TO NORMAL LIFE

You may be worried about carrying out your normal activities in the first few weeks or months after a heart attack, for example work or sexual activity.

DRIVING

You are usually not allowed by law to drive your car for one month after a heart attack. You do not need to notify the Licensing Authority, but you should probably tell your insurance company. There are special regulations for people who drive for their living, such as bus drivers and lorry drivers (LGV and PCV licence holders), and you should discuss these problems with your doctor. In some towns these regulations also apply to taxi drivers as well.

SEXUAL ACTIVITY

After a heart attack people worry about having sex. At first you don't usually feel like it but it is certainly reasonable to start sexual relations again 3–4 weeks after a heart attack if you want to. You should avoid being too vigorous until you feel fully recovered, which will normally be by about 6–8 weeks. Some of the drugs you may be taking can reduce sex drive and if you feel that this is the case you should have a word with your doctor.

WORK

After a heart attack most people can go back to work after 2–3 months. For those with a physically undemanding job that does not involve much exercise eight weeks off work may be enough. For heavy manual workers longer may be necessary and special exercises included in the exercise programme to build up your strength again. (Interestingly one of the first and most successful exercise programmes in Britain was in the Yorkshire town of Barnsley to help miners get back to work.)

HOLIDAYS

For the first 2–3 months after a heart attack it is probably safest not to go abroad. Later you can probably travel wherever you like provided you have made a full recovery. If in doubt, discuss your plans with your doctor. You should always make sure that you are fully insured and that the policy does not exclude a heart condition! If you are on medication, make sure you have enough to last while you're away, and keep them in your hand luggage.

— ANXIETY AND DEPRESSION —

Everyone worries after a heart attack and, despite all the positive advice from doctors, nurses and relatives, some people go on worrying. There is bound to be some concern about having another heart attack, and all that it entails. It's natural to be worried about yourself and your family, even if it's difficult to put into words exactly why. A heart attack can be a real blow to your self-confidence, especially if you have never had any serious health problems before, and it's relatively easy to become depressed.

GOING ON HOLIDAY
Once you have recovered from a heart attack long journeys are possible provided that you are fully insured and that you take the necessary medication with you.

RECOGNISING THE PROBLEM

Depression is just as much a real illness as heart disease, and also just as treatable. You may be depressed if you have several of the following symptoms:

- Sadness or tearfulness.
- Loss of enjoyment or interest in work and hobbies.
- Loss of interest in sex.
- Low self-esteem.
- Preoccupation with your health.
- Poor concentration.

- Sleep disturbance, difficulty getting to sleep or waking early.
- Constant tiredness.

In depression, the levels of chemicals that transmit signals to the brain are abnormally low and treatment with antidepressants can bring them back to normal. These drugs are not addictive, unlike tranquillisers, and you will be able to stop taking them once you have fully recovered from depression. Most people take them for at least 3–6 months.

In the first few weeks after a heart attack, there are so many things going on and so much to think about that depression may not be obvious. However, once things start to get back to normal, you may have more time to worry about the future, and this is when problems can occur.

The most common reaction is a short temper, even in people who have been quite placid, and partners often complain that they get their 'head bitten off' for the slightest thing. These problems usually settle down if and when the person returns to work, and life starts getting back to normal, but some people continue to have a 'short fuse' for much longer.

EXPERIENCING DEPRESSION
If you are suffering from depression, it is important to get help. Talking to others who have had the same experience may help.

The important thing about anxiety and depression is to realise that it is common and it can be helped. Often just discussing what you feel with someone else who has been through the same is all you need. Many towns now have a self-help group attached to the rehab service that gives long-term support where this is needed. If you have any of the symptoms listed on pp.77–78, don't just struggle on waiting for them to go, but consult your doctor.

KEY POINTS

- Most problems occur in the first 48 hours after a heart attack; after that life soon returns to normal.
- Regular exercise can help you to make a full recovery, but it should be supervised.
- Emotional problems after a heart attack are common and can be helped by talking about them and sometimes by drugs.

Looking after your heart

You may feel it is too late to think about prevention if you have already had a heart attack or developed angina. In fact, there are plenty of ways you can prevent the heart deteriorating further. There is a lot you can do to reduce your chances of having another heart attack by reducing your risk factors. This is especially important after bypass surgery as it means your new blood vessels will be less likely to fur up.

As we have already seen (pp.28–38), risk factors fall into two distinct categories: those over which you have no control and those that you can influence.

Other diseases, notably diabetes and hypertension (raised blood pressure), can increase the risk of developing CHD, but this risk is reduced if the conditions are well controlled with suitable medication.

REDUCING THE RISKS
Many factors contribute to heart disease. Some cannot be helped but others, such as a poor diet, can be changed.

LOWERING CHOLESTEROL

Lipids is the collective term used by doctors to refer to fat-like substances in the blood. Cholesterol is the best known, but another type called triglycerides also plays a role in CHD.

Cholesterol has a bad reputation as a cause of disease of the heart and blood vessels, but in fact it also performs some essential functions in the body and no one could do without it entirely. It is manufactured in the liver and is used in the cell membranes, to make bile and to form vital chemical messengers (or hormones). Therefore, even if you excluded cholesterol completely from your diet, you would always have some in your blood.

In practice, most diets in Western countries include large amounts of animal fat that the body converts into

Drugs for Raised Cholesterol

There are a number of drugs available to bring down the level of fat-like substances (known as lipids) in the blood.

DRUG GROUP	GENERIC NAMES	TRADE NAMES
Statins	Simvastatin	Zocor
	Pravastatin	Lipostat
	Fluvastatin	Lescol
	Atorvastatin	Lipitor
	Cerivastatin	Lipobay
Fibrates	Bezafibrate	Bezalip
	Gemfibrozil	Lopid
Resins	Colestipol	Colestid
	Cholestyramine	Questran

CHOLESTEROL TESTING
A simple blood test can provide an accurate measure of the amount of cholesterol in your blood.

cholesterol. These fats are absorbed by the stomach and intestines and passed to the liver, where they are broken down and circulated to the rest of the body to provide energy or to be stored in the fat cells. The fat circulates through the body in the blood in tiny particles containing mixtures of cholesterol and other fats.

When you have a blood cholesterol measurement, the laboratory will usually measure several other fats as well. The total cholesterol level is made up of two parts, called low-density lipoprotein (LDL) and high-density lipoprotein (HDL). LDL is the 'bad' cholesterol that, when the level is too high, builds up in the arterial wall to produce atheroma. About two-thirds of the cholesterol in the blood is LDL, and this is usually what doctors are referring to when they say you have a high cholesterol level.

HDL is, on the other hand, a 'good' cholesterol and the higher the level, the less likely you are to get heart disease. Women have a higher HDL level than men but this difference usually disappears after the menopause.

Triglycerides are the third type of fat measured in a blood sample. Triglycerides make up most of the fat in the fat cells of your body and, when released, provide the energy you need for everyday activities. Although triglycerides are not found in any quantity in the fatty deposits in arterial walls, high levels of triglycerides in the blood are indirectly linked to CHD.

Most people who have angina or a heart attack have high lipid levels, which are partly the result of what they eat and partly genetic. By careful dieting we can reduce lipid or cholesterol levels by 10–20 per cent but, if we want to lower them more than this, drugs are usually necessary.

You may find that your doctor prescribes more than one drug to lower lipids, as they work in different ways. However, you will also be given advice on reducing the amount of cholesterol in your diet as this is necessary if the drug treatment is to be fully effective (see pp.84–86).

STATINS

The big change in the treatment of cholesterol in the last five years has been the development of this new class of drug that works by slowing the production of cholesterol in the liver. Statins are able to lower cholesterol by 20–30 per cent and have very few side-effects.

There have now been several important studies, involving thousands of patients in Europe, Australia and the USA, showing that this reduction in cholesterol is followed by a 20–30 per cent reduction in the risk of further heart attacks. The most common statins used at present are simvastatin and pravastatin, although there are many more being released.

These drugs are usually taken as a single dose with the main meal of the day and have few side-effects. Very occasionally they may cause inflammation in the muscles of the arms and legs, an aching that feels like flu. This occurs in the first few weeks after starting treatment and should be reported immediately to your doctor. It settles once the tablets are stopped.

If you experience no problems with these drugs in the first few weeks of taking them, you are unlikely to develop any after that.

FIBRATES

For some individuals, particularly those with diabetes, the problem with the lipids may be not so much with cholesterol as with triglycerides, when another group of drugs called the fibrates may be used. Like the statins they have few side-effects and are taken with the main meal of the day. They too may produce muscular pains in the first few weeks but otherwise have few side-effects. They can reduce cholesterol levels by 10–15 per cent and cut the risk of CHD by about the same percentage.

RESINS

Resins reduce cholesterol levels by binding cholesterol in the intestines and affecting their absorption into the body. These are taken in the form of a powder, usually in fruit juice, once or twice a day. As they are not absorbed into the body, they cannot cause any serious side-effects in body tissues, but they can cause flatulence and belching or constipation in some people.

Resins too have been shown to reduce the risk of further heart attack, but they are less potent than the statins and reduce the risk by only 10–15 per cent.

IMPROVING THE DIET

Changing the sort of food that you have eaten all your life may not be easy but it is an important way to reduce the risk of further heart attack. The basic rules are fairly simple and given in the box on p.86.

Eating healthily doesn't mean giving up everything you enjoy or eating nothing but rabbit food. Most people consume far more fat, and especially animal or dairy fat, than is good for them and cutting down would be a health bonus for your whole family. Red meat, hard cheeses, butter, cream, full-fat milk and yoghurt as well as cooking fats such as lard are all high in so-called saturated fats, so it is wise to eat relatively little of them or just keep them for special occasions.

As well as reducing the overall amount of fat in your diet, you will do yourself a lot of good by using polyunsaturated fats – generally those from vegetable sources that are liquid at room temperature – or monounsaturated fat, such as olive oil, rather than animal (dairy) fat whenever you can. If you are not sure which are the healthy oils, check the label or ask a dietitian as one or two vegetable oils are not good for the heart. Coconut oil in particular is almost as bad for the heart as lard!

Cutting down on fats in general is a good way to lose weight, and many people find that, after changing their diet, they get much less indigestion. You may be concerned about your cholesterol levels and be anxious to avoid foods containing it, such as eggs, liver, kidney and shellfish. Although they do contribute some cholesterol, they are probably less important sources for most people than foods high in animal fats. It's worth bearing in mind too that many processed and prepared foods such as pies, biscuits, cakes and so on may be high in animal fats as, of course, are burgers! Now that we are all starting to become more health conscious, many foods in supermarkets are labelled to give us some idea of the fat content.

The other major change that will improve your diet from a health viewpoint is to eat as many pieces of fruit and vegetables as you can – at least five portions every day.

EATING WELL
A high-fibre diet, rich in fruit and vegetables, will benefit your overall health.

Four Steps to Healthy Eating

Anyone can eat more healthily by following these simple guidelines.

- Cut down the total amount of fat in your diet.
- Replace animal fats (including dairy fats) with vegetable oils.
- Eat more fresh fruit and vegetables.
- Go on a sensible weight-reducing diet if necessary.

If you can also increase your intake of other fibre-rich foods such as wholemeal bread, brown rice and pasta and breakfast cereals, especially oats, you will be well on the way to a diet that's good for your overall health as well as your heart.

Fortunately the food industry is beginning to realise the importance of a healthy diet, and there are also now many excellent recipe books to help. What many writers ignore, however, is the higher cost of some healthy foods, and this often puts a strain on the family budget. If this is a real problem you should discuss the matter with your family doctor. There may be benefits that you are entitled to, or a dietitian may be able to give you advice on the best way to budget the weekly shopping.

STOPPING SMOKING

The benefits of stopping smoking are real and start from the day you give up and, five years on, your risk of having another heart attack will be halved.

You do have to stop completely, however. Just cutting down or changing from cigarettes to cigars or a pipe does little to reduce the risk.

Doctors realised this 30 years ago when the research linking heart disease and smoking was first published. Until then, doctors were among the heaviest smokers, and now there are very few doctors who smoke.

Many people find it easy to stop smoking in hospital, but it's much harder to keep it up when you go home. If you have smoked since you were a teenager, it can be a real problem. This is where all the family can help, because there is nothing worse when the craving is there than for your partner or daughter to light up. Hospitals are now 'no smoking' areas and your home should be too!

What is the best way of giving up? That's going to be different for everyone. Some people have found it easiest to stop suddenly. Others prefer to stop gradually, perhaps cutting down by a cigarette a day over several weeks. Part of the problem is an addiction to nicotine itself, and for some the use of nicotine chewing gum or skin patches can be a great help.

Sometimes talking to others trying to give up is the best help, and many hospitals and health centres run 'stopping smoking' sessions. Some even swear by hypnosis – as doctors we don't care so long as you kick the habit!

One of the things that often puts people – especially women – off giving up smoking is the tendency to put on weight afterwards. We are still not sure why this happens. Certainly the appetite improves, and some people take to eating sweets to reduce their craving for a cigarette. On average most people put on between half and one stone in the first six months after stopping smoking. However, if you change to a healthier, low-fat diet at the same time the extra weight usually comes off again gradually over the next 6–12months.

REDUCING STRESS

When you develop angina or have had a heart attack, it is an opportunity to weigh up the priorities in your life. You may feel that a job that has occupied a large proportion of your time and energy over the years now seems less important to you than your family and friends and your other interests. Although there is no scientific

THE SMOKING FACTOR
Smoking greatly increases your risk of suffering from heart disease. However, if you give up smoking, your risk of CHD declines rapidly.

proof that changing the way you live reduces your risk, it will certainly improve the quality of your life.

PROTECTIVE FACTORS

Factors that are thought to offer some protection against coronary heart disease include a moderate alcohol intake and regular exercise.

ALCOHOL

There has been a lot of publicity recently about the good effects of alcohol when taken in moderation, but high levels of alcohol taken regularly can also poison the heart as well as the brain and the liver.

So what is moderation? The amount of alcohol that seems to be good for you is around 2–3 units a day, with women sticking to the lower end of the range. A unit is a measure of spirits, glass of wine or half a pint of beer or cider. Although it was first thought that red wine was particularly good at preventing heart attacks, it now seems that in fact any form of alcohol has the same effect.

EXERCISE

Regular exercise is also good for you and can protect against CHD. There have been many studies in the USA and Europe that show regular exercise (20 minutes, 2–3 times a week) reduces the risk of CHD when compared with the 'couch potatoes' of this world.

If you have actually had a heart attack, you will be taught about exercise in your rehabilitation sessions, but in fact anyone who has any form of CHD may well need more exercise too. If you have never exercised before and are unsure how to start, do ask your doctor's advice. The type of exercise you go for is probably not important

Recognising a Unit of Alcohol

Various drinks contain different amounts of alcohol. A unit of alcohol is equivalent to approximately 8–10 grams of pure alcohol.

WHAT IS A UNIT?
As different drinks contain different amounts of alcohol, alcoholic consumption is measured in units. Recommended intake is 2–3 units a day.

Small glass of sherry = 1 unit

Small glass of wine = 1 unit

½ pint of beer or cider, or ¼ pint of strong lager = 1 unit

Single measure of aperitif or spirit = 1 unit

A standard bottle of spirits (brandy, gin, whisky) = 30 units

providing it stimulates the heart and circulation sufficiently. You should do what you like best: walking, swimming, jogging, exercising in the gym or even dancing are all likely to help. Most people will need to start relatively slowly and build up to longer and more strenuous sessions gradually. If you go to a gym or an exercise class, you should be shown how to warm up properly beforehand, and it's a good idea to get into the habit of doing this with any exercise session.

The idea of 'going for the burn'– exercising until it hurts and beyond – has been thoroughly discredited. If you feel pain, dizziness or find it hard to breathe, stop and rest and have a break from exercise if you are injured or not feeling well.

— WORKING WITH YOUR DOCTOR —

Although smoking and lipid levels are major risk factors that are to a large extent under your own control, there are other spheres where you and your doctor will need to work together to minimise the risk of further problems. For one thing, people with conditions that make CHD more likely, such as diabetes and hypertension (high blood pressure), need to try and keep good control (see pp.34-37).

HYPERTENSION

Make a big effort to take your tablets regularly, even though you have no symptoms. See your doctor for regular blood pressure checks.

DIABETES

Try to keep your weight as close as possible to what it should be for your height.

Do your best to keep your blood glucose levels within the normal range by paying careful attention to your diet and taking your prescribed treatment properly. Exercise is important because it helps to reduce your weight and also reduces your insulin requirement.

RAISED LIPID LEVELS

Make an effort to stick to your diet and take any tablets prescribed correctly.

COPING IN AN EMERGENCY

A heart attack can happen anywhere and everyone should know what to do to help someone if they collapse and the heart stops beating. Basic life support (or BLS) is not difficult and it may literally be life saving to learn how to do it. Instructors are available in most towns, from voluntary agencies such as the St. John's Ambulance or from the local hospital.

If you or someone you are with develops chest pain that seems similar to the heart pain associated with an earlier heart attack, there are some basic steps to follow:

- Rest sitting or lying down.
- Take GTN medicine and wait for five minutes.
- If the pain is still as bad or worse after 5–10 minutes, take a second dose.
- If this has no effect, telephone for an ambulance.
- Chew on an aspirin (unless you or the person concerned is known to be allergic to it) as this will start to thin the blood and discourage clots.

KEY POINTS

- Changing to a healthy diet improves your fitness.
- Drug treatment to lower cholesterol reduces the risk of CHD.
- Stopping smoking reduces your risk further and is effective immediately.
- Regular exercise improves the state of your heart and circulation.

Emergency Tactics – ABC

In an emergency, it is important to check the ABC functions – airway, breathing and circulation.

AIRWAY
Ensure that there is nothing preventing air getting in through the nose and mouth.

BREATHING
See whether there is any spontaneous breathing.

CIRCULATION
Feel for a pulse in the neck.

If there is no breathing and you cannot feel the pulse, a cardiac arrest has probably occurred. Call for help and, if you know how, start mouth-to-mouth respiration and cardiac massage.

Useful addresses

British Cardiac Society
9 Fitzroy Square
London W1P 5AH
Tel: (0171) 383 3887

British Diabetic Association
10 Queen Anne Street
London W1M 0BD
General enquiries:
(0171) 323 1531
Careline: (0171) 636 6112,
Monday–Friday

British Heart Foundation
14 Fitzhardinge Street
London W1H 4DH
Tel: (0171) 935 0185

British Hypertension Society
127 High Street
Teddington
Middlesex TW11 8HH
Tel: (0181) 725 3412

Coronary Prevention Group
The London School
of Hygiene
Department of Public
Health and Policy
42 Store Street
London WC1E 7DB
Tel: (0171) 927 2125

Family Heart Association
7 North Road
Maidenhead
Berkshire SL6 1PL
Tel: (01628) 628638

Health Education Authority
Trevelyan House
30 Great Peter Street
London SW1P 2HW
Tel: (0171) 222 5300

The Resuscitation Council
5th Floor
Tavistock House North
Tavistock Square
London WC1H 9HR
Tel: (0171) 388 4678

Index

Acknowledgements

PUBLISHER'S ACKNOWLEDGEMENTS
Dorling Kindersley would like to thank the following for their help
and participation in this project:

Production Controller Michelle Thomas; **Consultancy** Dr. Sue Davidson;
Indexing Indexing Specialists, Hove; **Administration** Christopher Gordon.

Illustrations (p.15, 17, 41, 43, 55, 60, and 62) ©Gillian Lee;
(p.10, 21, 29, and 33) Passmore Technical Art Services

Picture Research Angela Anderson; **Picture Librarian** Charlotte Oster.

PICTURE CREDITS
The publisher would like to thank the following for their kind
permission to reproduce their photographs. Every effort has been made
to trace the copyright holders. Dorling Kindersley apologises for any
unintentional omissions and would be pleased, in any such cases,
to add an acknowledgement in future editions.

APM Studios p.89; **Sally & Richard Greenhill Photo Library** p.77; **Science Photo Library**
p.3 & 14 (Martin Dohrn/Royal College of Surgeons), p.46 (Simon Fraser), p.49 (CNRI),
p.50 (Matt Meadows), p.51 (Lunagrafix), p.53 and jacket (Simon Fraser), p.65 (Adam Hart-Davis),
p.68 (St.Bartholomew's Hospital); **Telegraph Colour Library** p.36